*What readers are saying about Heather Van Vorous's*

# Eating for IBS

"I have had yet another day of feeling great thanks to your tips. It's funny, I consider myself a healthy person. Yet none of that matters when you suffer from IBS. Knowing that I can really make a difference without feeling deprived by a strict diet is a wonderful feeling. The good news is that your tips will be easy for me to follow. That is half the battle right there! How does it feel to have made such a positive impact on peoples lives? Thanks again!"

—CINDY FRIEDMAN, IBS sufferer

"I just wanted to write and thank you for writing the best book on IBS that I have ever read. I have lived with IBS and lactose intolerance for twenty years with much confusing advice from my doctors about nutrition and diet. Your book puts everything into perspective for me. Not only is the information accurate; your recipes are absolutely fantastic. I now feel I can get off the deprivation diet and join my friends and family in eating healthy, normal, flavorful meals. Thank you so much. As a librarian, I have met several people who suffer from IBS and who come to the library to find information that will help ease their symptoms. Like myself, most of these people are frustrated by the lack of useful information out there or inaccurate information that they receive from both their physicians and from printed information resources. As I stated before, your book is the best and most accurate resource I have ever found. I will be happy to spread the word to as many people as I possible can. Thanks so much."

—PAIGE ANDERSON, IBS sufferer

"Your book has become my eating bible. Your advice has been better than that of my gastroenterologist's and two other books I've read. I feel so much better thanks to you. Your trail mix snack and rice pudding are life-savers as are many of your other recipes. Thanks again."

—JIL HAUGE, IBS sufferer

"We just found out that our son has IBS. He is ten years old and very scared and upset. Unbeknownst to my husband and me, his problem has gone on for a couple of years. He did not want to tell us. We feel like the worst parents in the world. Our doctor suggested your Web site and book. Thank you so much for this book. Now my son knows he is not alone."

—STACY AND ROBERT W., parents of IBS sufferer

"I am a forty-five-year-old woman who has suffered with IBS all of my life. I read all your information and made drastic changes in my diet and habits. It's been two weeks now, and for the *very* first time, I am feeling good. *Feeling good.* That is an amazing feeling. I have always thought most people took it for granted. I wanted to thank you. Your information has changed my life, and I do not say that lightly. Thank you!!!"

—BARBARA S. SAEGER, IBS sufferer

"I just wanted to let you know I bought your book a few weeks ago, and I carry it around like my little bible now. I bought a copy for my sister for her birthday, and we're ready to spread the word. It's such a great help, really, and all so logical. Thanks for having the energy and enthusiasm to write such a great cookbook for those of us with such touchy tummies."

—KAREN BAKER, IBS sufferer

"I recently purchased your book. I have just been diagnosed with IBS, and your book is such a wonderful help. I must have had IBS for years without realizing what it was; it's just increased in intensity in the last year or so. You have validated many of the strategies that I came upon by trial and error and just being in tune with my body. And you have given me so much more to help with this ailment."

—IRIS HURWITZ, IBS sufferer

"I just finished reading your book on IBS, and it is by far the most researched and informative book on IBS that I have read. Congratulations on your great work! Again, a warm *thank you* for being an advocate and educator for many!"

—JANET HALL, IBS sufferer

"Thank you! I've had IBS since I was nine (some of my earliest memories are of sitting in the back of a car in excruciating pain during family trips and not telling anyone). Reading your observations was like reading my own thoughts. I've learned from over forty years of trial and error what works for my diet and you are right on the money. Even if I didn't love to read and cook, I'd buy your book just to give you the support you deserve. The Web site is just terrific and serves you well. Keep it up and thank you again."

—G. Rivera, IBS sufferer

**HEATHER VAN VOROUS** has had IBS for more than twenty years, beginning in childhood. She is now a food writer specializing in healthy gourmet and ethnic recipes, with a special interest in cooking for people with bowel disorders. Her Web site, *www.eatingforibs.com*, has become the Internet's premiere source of IBS dietary information, and led directly to her first book, *Eating for IBS*. That work has received several thousand letters of accolade from readers and physicians alike, and generated many guest appearances on radio and television shows. She currently has a healthy cooking show in development for broadcast on both the Web (*www.heathercooks.com*) and cable access television stations. Heather now teaches classes on eating for IBS and works with corporate human resources departments to offer employee IBS education programs. She is a Seattle native who is happily at home in the Pacific Northwest.

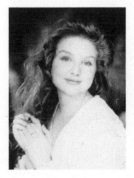

PHOTO©: MIKE DOUCETTE

THE FIRST YEAR®

# IBS

## (Irritable Bowel Syndrome)

# IBS

## (Irritable Bowel Syndrome)

*An Essential Guide for the Newly Diagnosed*

## Heather Van Vorous

Foreword by David B. Posner, M.D.

Da Capo
LIFE
LONG

A MEMBER OF THE PERSEUS BOOKS GROUP

Copyright © 2001 by Heather Van Vorous
Foreword copyright © 2001 by David B. Posner, M.D.

Designed by Pauline Neuwirth, Neuwirth and Associates, Inc.

Cataloging-in-Publication data for this book is available from the Library of Congress.

ISBN: 978-1-56924-547-7

Published by Da Capo Press
A Member of the Perseus Books Group
www.dacapopress.com

Da Capo Press books are available at special discounts for bulk purchases in the U.S. by corporations, institutions, and other organizations. For more information, please contact the Special Markets Department at the Perseus Books Group, 2300 Chestnut Street, Suite 200, Philadelphia, PA, 19103, or call (800) 810-4145, extension 5000, or e-mail special.markets@perseusbooks.com.

22  21  20  19

To the thousands of people with IBS
who have written me with questions,
comments, and suggestions, in
both desperation and gratitude.
This book is truly for you.

*And as always, for Will—with much love*

# Contents

# Your First Year: Learning From Living Every Month

# Foreword
By David B. Posner, M.D.

**IRRITABLE BOWEL** syndrome (IBS) is a common afflic-
tion. In fact, it is one of the most common causes of visits to
doctors in the United States. However, IBS does not get much
attention in the medical establishment. Many physicians tend
to minimize the illness, for several reasons. For one, there is
no medical test that can positively identify the condition;
rather, it is diagnosed when test results for conditions with
similar symptoms come out normal, and all other illnesses are
ruled out. Further, there is no risk of death from IBS, and
patients are rarely granted official disability status. Patients
are often misdiagnosed as psychosomatic or neurotic, and this
contributes to the fact that they do not receive the attention
patients with "real" diseases get.

Very few research dollars have been spent for this condition
in the past. Medical conferences tend to focus on exotic diseases that many practitioners see once or twice in a lifetime.
They often do not discuss common, everyday problems such
as this one. Treatment is generally unsatisfactory for many of
the patients because the symptoms are not always relieved,
and patients are left wondering what is going on in their bod-

ies, or if they are crazy. Sometimes a patient's symptoms are related to underlying problems that manifest in IBS complaints, and sometimes patients become depressed (for example) because of the chronicity of their complaints. These issues take a great deal of time to evaluate. The patients generally get short visits with their primary doctors that do not address the patients' complaints and concerns.

They do, however, have a real medical problem, with real symptoms. In her first book, *Eating for IBS,* Heather Van Vorous describes the dietary treatment of her symptoms and the diet therapy she adopted when she found conventional medical treatments were not successful in alleviating her symptoms. Now, in this book, she describes other practical ways of managing the disease, including ways of dealing with the stresses that can exacerbate the illness and the stresses that can result from the illness. She discusses alternative treatments such as hypnosis and acupuncture. Van Vorous has kept current on the research into the etiology and newest treatment modalities. She also suggests non-medical treatments such as the diet advice from her first book. She includes anecdotes from people she has corresponded with via the Internet. She provides practical and helpful advice that certainly can help many with the condition, and provides much-needed support for people frustrated with their condition.

Addressing Irritable Bowel Syndrome in a way such as this has been a long time coming. I think it will help me in my practice, and I would recommend it to physicians who see these patients, to provide them with another resource to suggest to their patients. I also believe that self-help is extremely important in the management of this disorder. If people who have IBS gain insight into this problem from reading this book, many of them will be better able to cope with the problems that the illness causes.

*DAVID B. POSNER, M.D., is a graduate of the California Institute of Technology and the University of Maryland School of Medicine. He is the Chief of Gastroenterology at the Mercy Medical Center in Baltimore, Maryland and holds a teaching appointment at the University of Maryland.*

# Introduction

**THIS IS** a book I never intended to write. After all, why would I? Why write anything about IBS when for the first twenty years I suffered from the disorder I never once met someone else with the same problem? IBS wasn't something I even talked about with friends, let alone a topic I envisioned myself becoming some sort of "expert" on. Just the thought conjured up awful visions along the lines of introducing myself with, "Hi, my name's Heather. And this...is my colon." Not exactly a glamorous path to fame and fortune. Embarrassment and isolation were more like it.

I honestly believe that, to this day, I still wouldn't have met another IBS sufferer had it not been for my first book, *Eating for IBS*. That book was as unexpected an event in my life as this one. It evolved from a two page e-mail letter I sent to people on IBS Internet boards into a full-fledged Web site, and only from there, in quite a roundabout manner, did it eventually end up as an actual published book. Over the long course of writing *Eating for IBS*, and since its publication, I have been overwhelmed with letters from other IBS sufferers desperate for help, answers, a sympathetic ear, and a little understanding from someone who could truly relate firsthand to the sheer misery they were enduring.

These letters raised issues outside the dietary aspects of IBS that begged to be addressed. People both newly diagnosed and longtime sufferers were asking the same questions. What is IBS? Why did I develop it? What are all the triggers, and why do attacks sometimes strike so unpredictably? Why doesn't anyone seem to take this problem seriously? Am I supposed to just live with IBS forever, and if so *how?*

As the letters piled up into the thousands (literally), the questions they asked began to weigh heavily on me. I started to consider writing a book that dealt with IBS in depth and addressed the full spectrum of ways to manage it. Having heard from so many people whose lives were transformed by the IBS dietary information alone, I realized that a broader book could surely accomplish even more. People were telling me that they were now able to drive, take vacations, hold a job, and socialize for the first time in years simply as a result of adopting the IBS diet. How much more dramatically could their lives be improved by comprehensive information about all IBS management strategies?

My own life offered a happy answer to this question, as the various elements required for successfully dealing with IBS on a daily basis have long been habitual for me, and are now ingrained to such an extent that I usually feel confident taking my good health and the freedom it allows for granted. To a great degree this is simply the end result of having had to deal with the disorder since I was nine years old. At that time I suffered my first attack, which struck out of the blue while I was playing in a neighbor's garden. The pain was so severe it quite literally took my breath away. I was unable to move or speak, and I eventually blacked out. When I recovered and made my way home, my parents took me to my pediatrician, who announced without running a single diagnostic test that my symptoms didn't fit any disorder she'd ever heard of. She refused to refer me to a gastroenterologist and told me to "quit whining." For years she dismissed my symptoms, ignored the fact that the attacks were so severe they sometimes woke me from a sound sleep in the middle of the night, and didn't even believe me when I told her I actually lost consciousness from the pain. It was seven long years later before I finally saw a doctor who was able to diagnose me, and by that time I had come to realize that while the attacks probably weren't going to kill me (though the pain did make me want to die), they were also not going to simply disappear (no matter how fervently I hoped and prayed). I desperately needed some help. Unfortunately, while my diagnosis did at long last give me a name for my problem, it didn't come with much information about what was physically wrong with me, and beyond a recommendation to use Metamucil I wasn't offered any advice at all about how to prevent or stop attacks.

Once again, I was left to deal with the pain all alone and try to find the answers to my questions, blindly hoping that if I just searched long and hard enough I would be able to successfully overcome the disorder through my own attempts. Though it was difficult and at times extremely frustrating, over the course of many years that's exactly what happened. The answers to my questions eventually came from twenty years of firsthand experience with countless trial-and-error discoveries, equally lengthy and ongoing research into applicable health and lifestyle issues, and extensive tracking of current scientific IBS findings. The answers I found form the chapters of this book.

My primary goal in writing *The First Year—IBS* has been to imagine the possibility of being transported back in time, so that I could give my younger self a guidebook for living with the disorder. What advice would have helped me then? What information and support did I need most? What exactly would I tell my nine-year-old self if I really could go back in time? The result is a sort of "survivor's manual" that details the strategies needed to control IBS on both a short and long term basis—and I can't tell you how much I wish I really could send this book through a time machine to make it available to me back when I so urgently needed it.

Dietary guidelines, strategies, and recipes are covered, and some of this information overlaps that in *Eating for IBS* as diet is truly a crucial means for managing IBS. But there is also comprehensive and empathetic information about stress management, suggestions for dealing with friends and family members, advice to enable you to work around the illness while learning to overcome it, and detailed coverage of alternative therapies that may well help more than prescription medications. There are also special sections throughout the book just for children with IBS and their parents, because they have unique concerns to be dealt with. These sub-chapters draw extensively from my own perspectives, experiences, and memories from childhood, and the issues they address remain very close to my heart.

Medical information is also given in detail, though, in general, physicians have had a poor track record when it comes to researching IBS (particularly in comparison to other chronic illnesses), and in fact very few studies were conducted until quite recently. As a result, there is much to be desired in how some medical professionals deal with this problem, and what they have to offer their IBS patients. Things are finally, fortunately, changing in this area, but it sure has been a long time coming. We're still nowhere near where we need to be in terms of medical solutions to what is indisputably a physical problem.

Personally, I simply couldn't wait for my doctors to get their acts together—I had to get mine together without them. IBS would have seriously compromised every single area of my life otherwise. So gradually, painfully, I did just that. And so can you—I promise. One of the most difficult aspects for me was feeling like I was all alone in the world with this problem, but you should never feel the same way. You are most definitely not alone. I realize now with hindsight that I actually had the power to successfully deal with IBS when I was nine—I just didn't have the information and knowledge required to do so. It took almost twenty years of learning and living to acquire that ability. Although I can't really send this book into the past to help myself, I am truly grateful that I can share what I've learned with the people who, unbeknownst to me until quite recently, have been struggling alongside me the whole time.

One of the fundamental tenets of this book, from day one through the end of your first year and beyond, is the idea that from this point forward you and your health must be a priority. You're worth it, so don't let anyone suggest otherwise. You will have to make time in your life to eat properly, exercise, manage your stress, try alternative therapies, and generally adjust your lifestyle to accommodate IBS by *preventing* the symptoms. There's something very important to note here—you're probably already living your life around IBS, but in terms of dealing with the symptoms. Planning extra time in the bathroom, driving an inconvenient route that allows quick access to restrooms along the way, avoiding restaurants and travel, minimizing social occasions where you have to eat—all of these restrictions and deprivations should end. You will still spend time planning, but to prevent problems, not accommodate them. The hours you've been wasting worrying about an attack, living in fear of one, or enduring one, will now be free. You will simply have to spend some of that time instead on a little daily lifestyle management to prevent the onset of attacks. This involves not just the avoidance of triggers, but taking active steps to maintain stable health on a continuous basis.

The calendar format of this book is well-suited to giving information about IBS in manageable segments (Learning), and throughout each chapter you'll be walked through ways to take this new knowledge and actually apply it to your life (Living). We'll start with a day-by-day guide to your first week that answers questions about what, exactly, IBS is, and how you can take control of the problem *immediately*. We'll then cover each subsequent week for your entire first month, and finally address each month for the rest of the year. As you progress into later chapters and grow habituated to the various IBS management strategies, the learning and living elements of the book will be smoothly combined. This shift will allow you to broaden your focus and continually expand your most personally successful means of controlling symptoms to further-reaching areas of your life. You will continue to learn as you follow the months, but there will be a gradual transition as your knowledge begins to come from experience itself, and your living techniques will both respond to and reflect this changing mindset.

This segue from discrete Learning and Living sections to a seamless integration of the two as the calendar progresses will support the evolution in your life from attack/response mode to an ingrained practice of continual symptom management, with a consistent emphasis on prevention and stability. This is an important point to note because it derives from three key ways in which IBS differs from most other chronic health problems.

First, IBS is not a disease, it's a disorder, and a historically neglected one at that. This means that while scientific literature on the subject is scarce (a bad thing), medical concerns such as progression of the disorder, related illnesses, surgical possibilities, and the development of serious complications are either strictly limited or simply nonexistent (a very good thing). The second unusual aspect of IBS is that, despite the fact that it's an extremely common disorder, most people suffer for years without receiving an accurate diagnosis. As a result, by the time someone is finally diagnosed they are often desperate for information, may well have turned to searching for answers on their own, and they not only want to know absolutely everything there is to know about the illness, they also want to know it all *right now*. They do not want information slowly parceled out to them, they don't want summary explanations, and they most definitely do not want to wait one extra minute for the knowledge they've been seeking for so long. The third critical element of IBS is that, in essence, when your GI tract is stable and you have no symptoms, you are no longer suffering from the syndrome. Though the underlying pathology that permits the symptoms to arise will still be present, IBS cannot exist in any relevant manner "in the background." Once your attacks are under control, you simply need to maintain the strategies that are working for you. You'll have no reason to give any further thought to IBS unless you're actually experiencing a flare. This is a radical difference from most other chronic illnesses (diabetes or high blood pressure, for example), where a person may feel fine but actually be suffering silent, serious physical damage unawares. With IBS, you simply can't have an attack and not know it (though don't we all wish!). Once your symptoms subside, for all intents and purposes you are no longer (albeit temporarily) living with IBS. Your goal is to make these "temporary" periods of stability last as long as possible. For me, that's now about ninety-nine percent of the time. My point of view is that I don't even have IBS outside of that one percent of my life. The daily symptom management strategies that I follow I consider to be for my overall good health, and not restrictions but benefits. I do not see myself as having a chronic illness because the vast majority of the time, I don't.

As a result of these three unique characteristics of IBS, you'll notice that this book provides in-depth information up front in the first seven days. This is so you can immediately take full advantage of the strategies you need to control your symptoms and run with them. Each approach for managing IBS will be visited at length early on, and then dealt with in their various tangents as you progress through the calendar. You'll seamlessly move from the core issues of symptom-control on a daily basis to expanding your lifestyle management abilities, gradually encompassing vacations, social events, support groups, and more.

Should you wish to follow your own pace and adjust the calendar stages to better fit your needs, please feel free. Skip ahead to future chapters if they're relevant to you now, skim the whole book initially before tackling each section in depth, or read each designated day, week, and month in strict order. The choice is yours. The structure of this book is meant only as a suggested means of managing the information you need to learn in order to live your life free from symptoms. It's important that you find a rate of progress you're comfortable with, whatever that may be.

I truly hope this book will be your shortcut to reaching a state of health, happiness, and confidence. May it give you the freedom to live your life however you choose, to go wherever you wish, whenever you want, and to eat, play, work, love, and laugh along the way. It took me almost two decades to get there, but then I had no one's help. Here's hoping that with this book you can reach that point well within your *First Year*. Good luck and good health to you!

## THE FIRST YEAR®

## IBS

(Irritable Bowel Syndrome)

*learning*

*task list*

> 1. **VERIFY THAT YOUR IBS DIAGNOSIS IS ACCURATE.**
>    - **DO YOUR SYMPTOMS MATCH THE CRITERIA?**
>    - **HAVE YOU HAD ALL THE NECESSARY MEDICAL TESTS?**
> 2. **LEARN THE PHYSICAL PATHOLOGY BEHIND YOUR SYMPTOMS.**

# You've Just Been Diagnosed with IBS. Now What?

**WELL, FIRST** of all, take a deep breath and try to relax. IBS is definitely not the end of the world. Make yourself a nice hot cup of peppermint or chamomile tea (both terrific GI muscle relaxants, and mint is packed with a pain-reliever as well), and take a small measure of comfort in finally knowing what's wrong with you. Odds are you've been wondering what the problem was for quite a while. The (only) great thing about IBS is that it is not associated with, nor does it lead to, any other illness. It will not progress, it does not raise your risk of colon cancer, it never requires surgery, and it is not a genetic disorder you can pass on to your children. Since IBS can be a god-awful problem in its own right, it's nice to know that at least you don't have anything else to worry about in the future. Once you learn how to control your symptoms, you've effectively solved the problem.

Second, take another deep breath, because you might not have been properly diagnosed after all. Unfortunately, there are a great number of much more serious GI tract problems that can mimic IBS, and many patients are given an IBS diagnosis before they have had all (or even any) of the tests required to eliminate other disorders. Before you accept a diagnosis of IBS, make sure that you have had the following problems conclusively ruled out:

colon cancer
inflammatory bowel diseases (Crohn's and ulcerative colitis)
bowel obstructions
diverticulosis
gallstones
food allergies
celiac (a genetic, autoimmune disorder resulting in gluten intolerance)
bacterial infections
intestinal parasites
endometriosis
ovarian cancer

What diagnostic tests does IBS require? Quite a few, and they're unpleasant but truly necessary. All possible physical, structural, and infectious abnormalities of the GI tract need to be unquestionably ruled out before you agree to an IBS diagnosis. This requires a physical examination, preferably by a board-certified gastroenterologist, and the following studies: complete blood count, sedimentation rate, and chemistries; stool for ova, parasites, and blood; urinalysis; liver function tests; rectal exam; abdominal x-rays; colonoscopy; for women, a gynecological exam including CA-125 blood test for ovarian cancer. Other diagnostic studies should be minimal and will depend on the symptom subtype. For example, patients with diarrhea-predominant symptoms should have a small bowel radiograph or lactose/dextrose H2 breath test. For patients with pain as the predominant symptom, a plain abdominal radiograph during an acute episode to exclude bowel obstruction and other abdominal pathology should be conducted. For patients with indigestion, nausea, and bloating, an abdominal ultrasound can rule out gallstones.[1] For patients with any numbness in association with constipation, Multiple Sclerosis should be excluded.

### FOR CHILDREN WITH IBS

*Children with IBS symptoms require fewer diagnostic tests than adults. Colon and ovarian cancers are not typical suspects, diverticulosis and gallstones are quite rare in childhood, and endometriosis does not occur in pre-pubescents. The remaining possible illnesses that can mimic IBS—particularly Crohn's, ulcerative colitis, and celiac—do need to be ruled out. It's worth noting that there is no doubt whatsoever that children can develop IBS, and there is no minimum age requirement for this disorder. I suffered my first attack at age nine; other children have been diagnosed as young as age three.*

## Had Your Gallbladder Out?

**IF YOUR** IBS symptoms are diarrhea-predominant, and began after you had your gallbladder or ileum (the last portion of the small intestine) removed, you are likely suffering from a malabsorption of bile acids secreted by the liver. These acids, which are normally stored in the gallbladder, are instead being dumped directly into the small intestines, causing chronic irritation and diarrhea. The prescription drug Questran (cholestyramine), which binds the bile acids in the intestines and prevents them from reaching the colon, can help this problem and should cure your "IBS." The bad news is you'll probably have to take Questran for the rest of your life. The good news is you don't need this book.

---

[1]Guidelines of the American Gastroenterological Association.

If you know you haven't had the proper tests for an IBS diagnosis, insist on them. If you're not sure whether or not you've had them, take this book into your doctor's office, have your chart pulled, and compare. If your doctor tells you all of these tests are unnecessary, say goodbye and find a new doctor.[2] I was diagnosed with IBS at the age of sixteen, ten years before I was actually given any of the tests necessary for a proper diagnosis. Had I actually had, say, a bowel obstruction instead of IBS, I could have died. Don't be as foolish as I was and accept a diagnosis without getting the tests to back it up. Your health and your life are on the line.

> *"I would have developed colon cancer and needed a colostomy, but my doctor told me I just had IBS."*
>
> —Ann G., Evansville, Indiana, age 53, misdiagnosed with IBS.

*"A few months ago I started feeling like I had hemorrhoids every day. My General Practitioner diagnosed me with IBS without running any tests, and prescribed medication. The pills did me little good and I was still miserable. One Sunday after a particularly uncomfortable day, I searched the Internet for information about IBS and found www.eatingforibs. com. I wrote the author of the site and told her my story, and she was very concerned when she learned that my symptoms began after age fifty. She urged me to have a colonoscopy. When I asked my GP about this he did not think my symptoms, or IBS in general, warranted it.*

*I made an appointment with another doctor to get a second opinion. He agreed I should have a colonoscopy, and thank goodness for this! During the colonoscopy the doctor found and removed a large benign polyp, which was quite extensive and would have become cancerous. I would have ended up with a colostomy. The doctor wants me to have a flexible sigmoidoscopy in six months to make sure there are no new growths. I am so thankful I took matters into my own hands*

---

[2]Eighty-seven percent of U.S. doctors admit that physicians need better education about IBS. (Citation from the largest, most comprehensive national survey ever conducted on IBS, July/August 1999, by Schulman, Ronca and Bucuvalas, Inc., funded by GlaxoWellcome.)

*and searched for information about IBS. I'm also very glad I didn't lis-
ten to my first doctor and that I insisted on having the tests necessary
for an accurate diagnosis. My symptoms have improved dramatically
since the polyp was removed, and now I don't think I ever even had IBS
in the first place."*

Just as you should insist on the necessary tests for a diagnosis, you
should also consider yourself misdiagnosed if your symptoms do not fit
the standard for IBS. This is defined as continuous or recurrent lower
abdominal pain or cramping (from mild to excruciating) in association
with altered bowel motility (diarrhea, constipation, or both).[3] Attacks may
strike suddenly at any time of day or night, and may even occasionally
(though not typically) wake you from a sound sleep. Gas and bloating are
common, but vomiting isn't (though it can occur due to nausea from the
pain). Upper GI symptoms are *not* a part of the syndrome. For women,
attacks are often associated with their menstrual periods, particularly if
they are prone to menstrual cramps.[4]

It's important to note that it is the *combination* of symptoms that characterizes IBS—constipation as a stand-alone problem should not be
diagnosed as IBS, nor should abdominal pain that comes without a
change in bowel movements. Passing blood, running a fever, swollen
extremities, and joint pain are *not* symptoms of IBS, and point to more
serious disorders.

## Serious? My problem is serious! How dare anyone suggest otherwise?

As infuriating as it is, and despite the fact that IBS is a *very* serious
problem to people who suffer from it, it really isn't treated as such by

---

[3] "Rome II Diagnostic Criteria for Irritable Bowel Syndrome," *Gut* 45, Supplement II
(1999).
[4] The excess prostagladins associated with uterine cramps can also trigger gastrointestinal
spasms, with resulting pain and diarrhea.

many doctors, medical researchers, and the general public.[5] You may even have friends and family dismiss your problem as "all in your head." It's up to you to educate these people, and then dump them if they persist in their ignorance at the expense of your health. You deserve support, concern, and consideration for your problem. IBS may not be "serious" in that it will not kill you, but an attack can be so painful you wish you'd die just to end it. And that's pretty damn serious.

---

[5]A UCLA survey of approximately three thousand respondents illuminated how IBS had a strong negative effect on patients' quality of life:
   a. 40% reported intolerable abdominal pain
   b. 65% plan their day-to-day schedule based on the anticipated use of bathroom facilities
   c. 53% of patients with IBS declared that their health limited their activity whereas only 26% of individuals without IBS felt the same way.
In contrast, the majority of doctors interviewed about IBS underappreciated the seriousness of the condition, and 33% mistakenly believed that IBS was primarily a psychological problem.

*living*

# Inform Yourself

**OKAY, YOU** really, really do have IBS. Now what? Take another deep breath, find a mirror, and take a good long look at the only person in the world who can control the problem. IBS is considered a patient-managed illness, with good reason. There's frankly not a darn thing anyone else can do to control your symptoms. It's all up to you. You're going to have to make some adjustments to your life—probably major ones—in order to manage your IBS. Don't be scared. This is good news. You alone have the power to get and keep yourself healthy, and no one can take that away from you. All you truly need is information and support. So here we go.

## Information: Know the enemy

You now know that you have IBS, but what exactly does this mean? Irritable Bowel Syndrome (such a glamorous name, isn't it?) has been under-researched for decades, but that is finally changing. Over the past few years a great deal of new information regarding the brain-gut interaction that results in IBS has evolved, and more discoveries are being made all the time.[6]

First of all, realize that you are not alone. IBS is estimated to affect fifteen to twenty percent of all Americans, primarily (but certainly not exclusively) women. This is at least thirty-five million Americans, and half of them have never even seen a physician for their symptoms. Despite this, IBS is still the most frequently seen illness by gastroenterologists, and is one the top ten diagnoses among *all* U.S. physicians.[7] It is also, incredibly, the second leading cause of worker absenteeism (behind only the common cold).[8] These are pretty amazing statistics for a disorder that many people have never even heard of.

Interestingly, because IBS is a "functional" disorder, you can't actually be tested for it. Rather, it is determined by a diagnosis of exclusion. This is because there are no structural, inflammatory, biochemical, or infectious abnormalities present in IBS. In other words, when IBS patients are examined by doctors, there is no physical problem to be found. So, are you just imagining your symptoms? No—you absolutely are not. A functional disorder simply means that the problem is an altered physiological function (that is, the way your body works), rather than something that has an identifiable origin behind it. In other words, while an IBS attack and its resulting symptoms are clearly visible as physical manifestations, the underlying cause behind these symptoms is not. The root of the problem in IBS sufferers cannot yet be identified by yielding a positive result from any existing medical tests. What then, precisely, is wrong with the way your body works if you have IBS? Get ready....

## The brain-gut interaction

It can be difficult (and until recently, it was downright impossible) to find explicit scientific explanations for the precise bodily mechanisms behind IBS. Because this information is still limited in its availability, and because

---

[6] It can be helpful and just plain interesting to follow the research studies for IBS, and the best way to do this is through the internet. The largest IBS site online is *www.helpforibs.com/messageboards/*—all current news related to IBS research is posted here.

[7] American Gastroenterological Association.

[8] Citation from largest, most comprehensive national survey ever conducted on IBS, July/August 1999, by Schulman, Ronca, and Bucuvalas, Inc., funded by GlaxoWellcome.

many people with IBS are given cursory explanations of the disorder without also being handed resources permitting more in-depth research, I'm including a full technical discussion of IBS physiology. If this is beyond the pale for you, please feel free to skip ahead to the next page and the plain-English translation. Otherwise, read on.

The most recent evaluation model for IBS patients states that the symptoms of the disorder result from the neurologic enervation of the gastrointestinal tract, associated with altered interpretation of neurologic messages from the GI tract by the central nervous system. Input to the central nervous system from the gastrointestinal tract arrives at several different parts of the brain which are associated with interpretation and modulation of pain perception. Neurologic output from these areas are then returned to the gastrointestinal tract via the spinal cord. This circuit (from gut to brain and brain to gut) appears to be abnormal in patients with Irritable Bowel Syndrome, though the exact abnormalities remain unclear.[9]

Visceral (gut) pain in IBS is associated with increased prefrontal cortex activation in the brain. The normal correlation between subjective pain intensity and activation of the anterior cingulate and insula cortices of the brain is lost in IBS. Altered visceral perception, via changes in reflex responses and viscerosomatic referral areas, is common in IBS. Both hyperalgesia (lower pain threshold) and allodynia (pain perceived in non-sensory pathways) are involved in the development of visceral (gut) hypersensitivity. It is believed that, as a result of central sensitization, a sensory memory response is created, which exaggerates and prolongs subsequent stimulation. The pathophysiology of this visceral hyperalgesia (lower pain threshold in the gut) is incompletely understood and appears to stem from multiple factors.[10] Interestingly, although people with IBS show this visceral hypersensitivity, their peripheral pain thresholds are normal or even elevated in comparison to healthy individuals.[11]

---

[9] Front Range Gastroenterology Associates, P.C., Longmont, CO.

[10] *CME Monograph I: Functional GI Disorders IBS at a Glance: Nosology, Epidemiology, Pathophysiology.* American Digestive Health Foundation.

[11] Whitehead W.E., et al. "Tolerance for Rectosigmoid Distention in Irritable Bowel Syndrome." *Gastroenterology* 98 (1990): 1187–1192.

Neuro-imaging has actually provided direct evidence of physiological differences between normal individuals and those suffering from IBS in the way a visceral (gut) stimulus is processed in the brain.[12] PET scans show pronounced differences in the activation of certain parts of the brain relating to perception and pain in IBS patients versus normal individuals. MRI scans have demonstrated comparable results.

## Okay, in plain English, what does all this mean?

Clearly, it means that IBS is indisputably a physical problem. Simply put, the brain-gut interaction of people with IBS influences their bowel pain perception and motility. In a nutshell, the processing of pain information within the central nervous system varies between normal individuals and those of us with IBS, with the result that we can experience even normal GI contractions as painful. The interactions between our brains, central nervous systems, and GI tracts are just not functioning properly. We have colons that react to stimuli that do not affect normal colons, and our reactions are much more severe. The end result is heightened pain sensitivity and abnormal gut motility, in the form of irregular or increased GI muscle contractions. It is this gut overreaction and altered pain perception that cause the lower abdominal cramping and accompanying diarrhea and/or constipation that characterize IBS. Lucky us.

Interestingly, the origins of IBS may really be in our brains, and not in our bowels. Given that for many years people with IBS were dismissively told their problem was "all in their heads," it's ironic that, in the end, this may be factually true. The underlying problem might well be in our brains—but it's absolutely *not* in our imaginations.

Why are we the chosen not-so-few? No one really yet knows exactly why some people develop IBS and others don't. There is mounting evidence that for some IBS sufferers the condition is precipitated by some type of grievous insult to the gut—dysentery, food poisoning, intestinal flu, abdominal surgery, even pregnancy. The theory goes that even after

---

[12] Silverman D.H., et al. 1997. "Regional Cerebral Activity in Normal and Pathological Perception of Visceral Pain." *Gastroenterology* 112 (1997): 64–72.

Mertz H., et al. "Regional Cerebral Activation in Irritable Bowel Syndrome and Control Subjects with Painful and Nonpainful Rectal Distention." *Gastroenterology* 118 (1997): 842–848.

full physical recovery from these traumatic events, the nerves within the gut retain a "memory" of the insult and remain hypersensitive to further stimulation, as well as prone to subsequent overreaction. You likely know if you experienced any abdominal trauma immediately prior to the onset of your IBS symptoms, and if you did it's probably nice to have a logical explanation for what has happened to your GI tract and why. There are those of us who are exceptions to this theory, however, who suffered no gut injury prior to the onset of IBS symptoms, and we're still patiently waiting for our explanation.

**IN A SENTENCE:**

*Although IBS is a functional disorder of the GI tract and not a disease, it is a physical problem with serious and even debilitating symptoms. You need and deserve information, support, and consideration to deal with it.*

*learning*

*task list*

1. LEARN HOW YOUR GI TRACT SHOULD NORMALLY FUNCTION, AND WHAT'S GOING WRONG WITH IT WHEN YOUR IBS SYMPTOMS FLARE.

2. RECOGNIZE THE STRATEGIES THAT WILL BE KEY TO MANAGING YOUR HEALTH: PROPER DIET, CONTROLLING STRESS, TAKING MEDICATIONS, TRYING ALTERNATIVE THERAPIES, AND USING SUPPLEMENTS.

3. BE PREPARED TO TRY EACH MANAGEMENT STRATEGY IN TURN, AS WELL AS A COMBINATION OF ALL OF THEM.

# The GI Tract and How It (Should) Work

THE DIGESTIVE system is a series of hollow organs joined in a long, twisting tube from the mouth to the anus. Inside this tube is a lining called the mucosa. In the mouth, stomach, and small intestine, the mucosa contains tiny glands that produce juices to help digest food. There are also two solid digestive organs, the liver and the pancreas, which produce juices that reach the intestine through small tubes. In addition, nerves and blood play a major role in the digestive system.

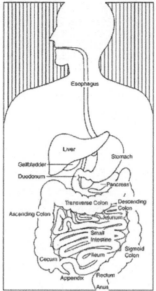

Figure 1. The Digestive System. Courtesy of the National Digestive Diseases Information Clearinghouse.[13]

Food, as it is eaten, is not in a form that the body can use as nourishment. It must be changed into smaller molecules of nutrients that can be absorbed into the blood and carried to cells throughout the body. Digestion is the process by which food is broken down into its smallest parts so that the body can use it to build and nourish cells and to provide energy. Digestion involves the mixing of food, its movement through the digestive tract, and the chemical breakdown of the large molecules of food into smaller molecules. Digestion begins in the mouth, with chewing and swallowing.

---

[13]The National Digestive Diseases Information Clearinghouse (NDDIC) is a service of the National Institute of Diabetes and Digestive and Kidney Diseases (NIDDK). The NIDDK is part of the National Institutes of Health under the U.S. Public Health Service. Established in 1980, the clearinghouse provides information about digestive diseases to people with digestive disorders and to their families, health care professionals, and the public. NDDIC answers inquiries; develops, reviews, and distributes publications; and works closely with professional and patient organizations and Government agencies to coordinate resources about digestive diseases.

Two types of nerves help to control the action of the digestive system. Extrinsic (outside) nerves come to the digestive organs from the brain or from the spinal cord, and they trigger the release of the chemicals acetylcholine and adrenaline. Acetylcholine causes the muscles of the digestive organs to squeeze with more force, and increases the transit speed of matter through the digestive tract. Adrenaline relaxes the muscles of the stomach and intestine and decreases the flow of blood to these organs.

Intrinsic (inside) nerves, which make up a very dense network embedded in the walls of the esophagus, stomach, small intestine, and colon, are triggered to act when the walls of the hollow digestive organs are stretched by food. In this regard they are rather like the strings of a musical instrument, which will play different notes depending on their tension. The varying tension levels of the intrinsic nerves trigger similarly varying reactions. Instead of sounding different notes they release many different substances, and either speed up or delay the movement of food and the production of juices by the digestive organs. As you can guess, the key roles of these extrinsic and intrinsic nerves in the GI tract help explain why stress has such a powerful effect on the digestive tract, and thus IBS. (I'll have more to say about this in Day 5.)

The hollow organs of the digestive system, such as the stomach and colon, contain muscles that enable their walls to move. The movement of organ walls can propel food and liquid and also can mix the contents within each organ. Typical movement of the esophagus, stomach, and intestine is called **peristalsis**. The action of peristalsis looks like an ocean wave moving through the muscle. The muscle of the organ produces a narrowing and then propels the narrowed portion slowly down the length of the organ. These waves of narrowing push the food and fluid in front of them through each hollow organ.

The first major muscle movement occurs when food or liquid is swallowed. Although beginning to swallow is a voluntary action, once the swallow begins it becomes involuntary and proceeds under control of the nerves. The esophagus is the organ into which the swallowed food is pushed. It connects the throat above with the stomach below. At the junction of the esophagus and stomach, there is a ring-like muscle that closes the passage between the two organs. However, as the food approaches the closed ring, the muscle relaxes and allows the food to pass. The food then enters the stomach, which has three tasks to do. First, the stomach must store the swallowed food and liquid. This requires the muscles of the upper part of the stomach to relax and accept large volumes of swallowed material. The second job is to mix the food and liquid with digestive juices, and this is what the lower part of the stomach does. The third task of the stomach is to empty its contents slowly into the small intestine.

Several factors affect emptying of the stomach, including the nature of the food (mainly its fat and protein content) and the degree of muscle action of the emptying stomach and the next organ to receive the stomach contents (the small intestine). As the food is digested in the small intestine, the contents of the intestine are mixed and pushed forward in the GI tract.

Finally, almost all of the digested nutrients are absorbed through the intestinal walls. The waste products of this process are undigested parts of the food, including soluble and insoluble fibers, and older cells that have been shed from the mucosa. These materials are propelled into the colon, which extracts any available nutritional material the small intestine was unable to collect. The colon is also where the reabsorption of water, electrolytes, and bile salts occurs, and contents are solidified into solid waste. The colon stores the waste products in the form of feces, usually for a day or two. If the waste products move too slowly through the colon, too much water is absorbed and the stool becomes hard and dry, with constipation resulting. If the material passes through the colon too quickly, not enough water is absorbed and diarrhea results.

The majority of the time the colon is still, barely moving a muscle. However, following a meal, the stomach triggers something called the **gastrocolic reflex**. This response occurs when food passes from the stomach into the upper part of the small intestine. Normally, the gastrocolic reflex causes periodic contractions of the colon at different points along its length, at timed intervals. These segmented contractions regulate the flow of waste, and keep it in contact with the bowel wall, allowing water to be absorbed.

Finally, peristaltic contractions of the colon propel the waste to the rectum and then out of the anus via evacuation by a bowel movement. Total average transit time through the entire thirty-foot digestive system, from mouth to anus, is 12–24 hours for healthy individuals with high-fiber diets, and 48–72 hours for most Americans eating a typical Western (high fat/protein, low fiber) diet.

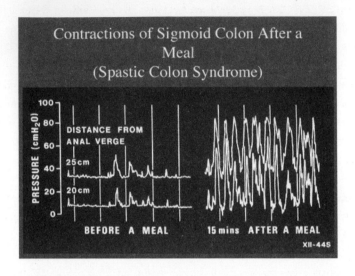

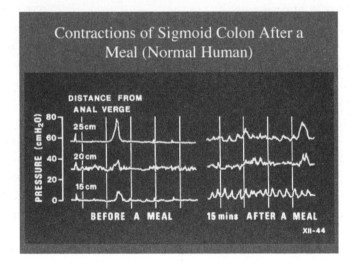

Figures 2 and 3. Illustrations from *Irritable Bowel Syndrome (IBS): Examining New Findings and Treatments*, Marvin M. Schuster, M.D.; Michael D. Crowell, Ph.D.; Nicholas J. Talley, M.D., Ph.D., Continuing Medical Education Activity, Johns Hopkins School of Medicine, via Medscape (October 26, 2000). Used by permission.

**THESE IMAGES** vividly demonstrate the difference between the after-meal contractions of a normal person's lower (sigmoid) colon and the contractions of the lower (sigmoid) colon in a person with IBS. The left half of both illustrations shows the colon contractions before a meal, and the rates are very similar and quite modest. Just fifteen minutes after eating, however, the differences in colon contractions as shown on the right sides of the graphics are dramatic. Given the almost off-the-chart severity of the spasms (measured by the vertical axis in terms of pressure) in the IBS patient, it's easy to literally see exactly why the pain and bowel dysfunctions of this disorder can be so extreme.

As you read these graphics, don't be intimidated by the "distance from **anal verge**" legend for the horizontal axis of the chart. All that term basically means is how far up into the colon from the anus the contractions are being measured (they're either fifteen, twenty, or twenty-five centimeters up into the colon from the outside of the anus). In other words, the contractions triggered by the gastrocolic reflex from the stomach are affecting the very lower end of the colon only fifteen minutes after a meal has been eaten. This gives a crystal-clear explanation for just how an attack can hit you so fast and so hard after—or even while—eating.

Personally, I can't look at these charts without having flashbacks to all the times I've had to rush from the dinner table before I've even finished my meal. The worst memory of all is from a vacation in Hawaii when I was twelve, and had been allowed to order a whole lobster for myself. Unfortunately, a virgin piña colada (in hindsight, it was the high-fat coconut milk on an empty stomach that did me in) triggered an attack before my meal had even arrived at the table. I spent the entire evening doubled over in agony in a bright pink hotel ladies lounge while my family ate my lobster. It's not much consolation to finally get a scientific explanation for exactly what happened to me that night, but I suppose it's nice to no longer be completely in the dark. And in case you're wondering, I haven't had a piña colada since.

## *Where things go wrong...*

Unfortunately, how the digestive tract is *supposed* to work is not exactly how it *does* work for those of us with IBS. The key problem seems to be with the gastrocolic reflex. Specifically, research has found that many IBS patients have highly abnormal ones.[14] Our colons have disorganized and significantly more violent and prolonged contractions (leading to diarrhea), or almost no contractions at all (resulting in constipation). Amazingly, researchers have found that while healthy people have six to eight peristaltic contractions in their colon within a twenty-four-hour period, IBS sufferers with diarrhea have as many as twenty-five peristaltic contractions per day, and constipation-prone IBS patients have almost none.[15] Add to this bowel dysfunction the heightened pain perception resulting from our abnormal brain-gut interactions, and you've got the recipe for disaster . . . spelled I-B-S.

---

[14] Constipation-predominant IBS is characterized by postprandial rectal relaxation, blunted gastrocolic response, and lower rectal discomfort threshold. Diarrhea-predominant IBS is characterized by a postprandial increase in rectal tone, an enhanced gastrocolic response, and hypersensitivity to rectal distention. [Schuster, Marvin M., M.D.; Michael D. Crowell, Ph.D; and Nicholas J. Talley, M.D., Ph.D. "Irritable Bowel Syndrome (IBS): Examining New Findings and Treatments." Continuing Medical Education Activity, Johns Hopkins School of Medicine, via Medscape (26 October 2000).]
[15] Hendricks, Melissa. "Bowels in an Uproar." *Johns Hopkins Magazine,* April 1997.

*living*

# Lifetime Lifestyle Management— The Five Key Strategies For Symptom Control

**YOU NOW** know that you do not have a properly functioning GI tract, you have an idea of what's physically going wrong, and hopefully you have a grasp of the underlying reasons why. Well, this knowledge is very nice and all, but the real issue is, *what can you do about it?* Fortunately, lots!

Diet and stress are typically the two greatest triggers of an abnormal gastrocolic reflex in people with IBS. Eating properly, managing stress, taking medications, trying alternative therapies, and using supplements are the five greatest weapons we have to keep our GI tracts functioning normally and thus prevent our symptoms. You might need to use just one approach, a combination, or all of them.[16] It will probably take a little trial-and-error experience to see what helps you the most, but fortunately there are some lifestyle changes you can make today that should be of immediate benefit. Other strategies may take a few weeks or months to help you significantly.

Personally, I've found benefits from all approaches except alternative therapies, which I haven't yet had much luck with though I know many others have. I've also learned that I need to approach my IBS management from both a day-to-day standpoint and with a continuous long-term view as well. To keep myself stabilized on a daily basis I rely primarily on an IBS-safe diet and peppermint tea, buttressed as needed with soluble fiber supplements. My second-line defense is prescription drugs, which I turn to when my daily management just isn't doing enough to prevent attacks, typically as a result of stress. I don't have to resort to medications too often, though, most likely because of ongoing stress management strategies that are always "in the background" of my daily life. For me the most effective means of preventing stress from triggering IBS are sleep, exercise, and reading (which has been my form of meditation since childhood, and is a necessity in my daily life in order to truly relax).

## Five Key Strategies to Control IBS

1. Diet (low fat, high soluble fiber, careful with insoluble fiber, avoid triggers)
2. Stress Management (exercise, sleep, meditation, yoga, Tai Chi)
3. Prescription Medications (anti-spasmodics, anti-depressants, opioids)
4. Alternative Therapies (hypnotherapy, acupuncture)
5. Supplements (soluble fiber, herbal teas, enzymes, calcium)

---

[16] Most IBS patients report relying on significant trial and error to treat their particular mix of symptoms. Various combinations of diet, stress management, alternative therapies, and medications allow them to arrive at a solution that works best for them. (Results from DrugVoice's IBSVoice survey of over two thousand patients, one of the largest and most far-reaching studies of IBS patients ever conducted. [Krauth, Melissa, President, DrugVoice LLC. Update on IBSVoice Panel (23 February 2001).]

You might want to begin by trying each approach to managing your IBS symptoms in turn, and deciding as you learn and live which particular strategies end up working best for you. So, let's take them in order beginning with Day 3.

**IN A SENTENCE:**

> *Eating properly, using supplements, managing stress, trying alternative therapies, and taking medications are the five best ways to keep your GI tract functioning normally. You may need to use just one approach, a combination, or all of them.*

# DAY **3**

*learning*

*task list*

1. **UNDERSTAND HOW CATEGORIES OF FOODS—FATS, INSOLUBLE FIBER, SOLUBLE FIBER—PHYSICALLY AFFECT YOUR GI TRACT.**

2. **BEGIN TO PRACTICE MENTALLY CATEGORIZING ALL THE FOODS YOU EAT SO THIS ABILITY BECOMES SECOND NATURE.**

3. **MEMORIZE AND FOLLOW THE 10 COMMANDMENTS OF EATING FOR IBS.**

# Food— Friend or Foe?

**YOU'VE JUST** learned exactly what happens to your colon, via the gastrocolic reflex, when you eat. I would bet you already know from personal experience that some foods nearly always cause problems, while others never seem to bother you. On the other hand, you've also probably noticed that sometimes a specific food will trigger an attack, while at other times you can eat the exact same item without difficulty. Odds are it doesn't seem like there's any rhyme or reason to this. Odds are also that you've been wracking your brain to figure out why.

There are, in fact, very clear guidelines to follow for how to eat safely for IBS, based on the well-established effects certain categories of foods have on the GI tract. The key word here is *categories*—most people with IBS drive themselves bonkers trying to find that one specific food that is triggering their attacks. The problem is, it isn't a single food that causes attacks. It's *any* food that is high in **fat**, *insoluble* **fiber, caffeine, coffee (even decaf), carbonation, or alcohol**. Why? Because all of these food categories are either GI stimulants or irritants, and can cause violent over-reactions of the muscles in your colon.[17]

## Soluble fiber—The good guy

Hmmm…. You've heard of fiber, you're pretty sure you know what it is, and you've probably had it recommended to you as beneficial for IBS. But *soluble* fiber? Is this something special?

Yes, it is. Soluble fiber is the single greatest dietary aid for preventing IBS symptoms in the first place, as well as relieving them once they occur. Here's the kicker. Soluble fiber is *not* typically found in foods most people think of as "fiber," such as bran or raw leafy green vegetables. Soluble fiber is actually found in foods commonly thought of as "starches," though soluble fiber itself differs from starch as the chemical bonds that join its individual sugar units cannot be digested by enzymes in the human GI tract. In other words, soluble fiber has no calories because it passes through the body intact.

---

[17]Comprehensive dietary information, eating and cooking strategies, travel and restaurant advice, daily menus, supermarket ideas, and one hundred seventy-five safe gourmet recipes for IBS can be found in *Eating for IBS*, by Heather Van Vorous (Marlowe & Company, 2000).

# Soluble Fiber Foods—
# The Basis of the IBS Diet

AS A general rule, the grain and cereal foods at the top of this list make the safest, easiest, and most versatile soluble fiber foundations for your meals and snacks.[18]

Rice

Pasta and noodles

Oatmeal

Barley

Fresh white breads such as French or sourdough (*not* whole wheat or whole grain. Please choose a baked-daily, high quality, preservative-free brand. White bread does not mean Wonder.)

Rice cereals

Flour tortillas

Soy

Quinoa

Corn meal

Potatoes

Carrots

Yams

Sweet potatoes

Turnips

Rutabagas

Parsnips

Beets

Squash and pumpkins

Chestnuts

Avocados (though they do have some fat)

Bananas

Applesauce

Mangoes

Papayas (also digestive aids that relieve gas and indigestion)

---

[18] Unfortunately, starchy foods are the enemies in the current high protein/low carbohydrate fad diets. Please realize that an overwhelming number of research studies on the subject consistently show that the healthiest diets in the world, across all countries and cultures, are those high in complex carbohydrates and low in fat and protein (particularly from animal products). For numerous resources and references in this area, please consult the Physician's Committee for Responsible Medicine. Founded in 1985, the PCRM is a nonprofit organization supported by over five thousand physicians nationwide, dedicated to promoting preventive medicine. PCRM—5100 Wisconsin Ave., Suite 400, Washington, D.C. 20016. Phone: 202-686-2210. *www.pcrm.org*.

Why is soluble fiber so special? Because unlike any other food category, it soothes and regulates the digestive tract, stabilizes the intestinal contractions resulting from the gastrocolic reflex, and normalizes bowel function from *either* extreme. That's right—*soluble fiber prevents and relieves both diarrhea and constipation.* Nothing else in the world will do this for you. How is this possible? The "soluble" in soluble fiber means that it dissolves in water (though it is not digested). This allows it to absorb excess liquid in the colon, preventing diarrhea by forming a thick gel and adding a great deal of bulk as it passes intact through the gut. This gel (as opposed to a watery liquid) also keeps the GI muscles stretched gently around a full colon, giving those muscles something to easily "grip" during peristaltic contractions, thus preventing the rapid transit time and explosive bowel movements of diarrhea as well. By the same token, the full gel-filled colon (as opposed to a colon tightly clenched around dry, hard, impacted stools) provides the same "grip" during the muscle waves of constipation sufferers, allowing for an easier and faster transit time, and the passage of the thick wet gel also effectively relieves constipation by softening and pushing through impacted fecal matter. If you can mentally picture your colon as a tube that is squeezing matter through via regular waves of contractions, it's easy to see how a colon filled with soluble fiber gel is beneficial for both sides of the IBS coin.

As a glorious bonus here, normalizing the contractions of the colon (from too fast or too slow speeds) prevents the violent and irregular spasms that result in the lower abdominal cramping pain that cripples so many IBS patients. This single action alone is the reason I don't eat anything on an empty stomach but soluble fiber. Ever. The only foods I want to trigger my gastrocolic reflex are soluble fiber, because that's the only way I can keep those contractions (and thus my life) normal. I routinely snack on small quantities of sourdough bread, rice cakes, homemade quick breads (pumpkin, zucchini), bananas, baked corn chips, and so on, all day long, every single day. If I don't have a chance to eat or I'm not that hungry, I'll take some Fibercon tablets or a glass of Metamucil (these are both soluble fiber supplements—*not* laxatives—and are dealt with in depth in Month 2). My goal is continual stability, and a steady ingestion of soluble fiber ensures this. In the short run this strategy

# Danger—High Fat Foods Ahead

**PLEASE DON'T** read this list and assume that you can never again eat any of these foods, so life is no longer worth living. These are all triggers, yes, and some of them you will probably have to completely eliminate from your diet. *But—* others can be eaten in small quantities when you follow the Day 3 Living guidelines coming up, many of the items listed have safer substitutes you can use freely, and there are quite a few tips and tricks you'll soon learn for cooking with the nutritious foods on the list in a safe manner. So take heart, this isn't the end of the world—it's just the beginning of a better diet.

**Red meat** (ground beef, hamburgers, hot dogs, steaks, roast beef, pastrami, salami, bologna, pepperoni, corned beef, ham, bacon, sausage, pork chops, and anything else that comes from cows, pigs, sheep, goats, deer, etc. )

**Poultry dark meat and skin** (the white meat is fine, as is seafood by the way—try to buy organic turkey and chicken)

**Dairy products**[19] (cheese, butter, sour cream, cream cheese, milk, yogurt, cream, half and half, ice cream, whipped cream). *Even skim and lactose-free dairy can trigger IBS attacks. In addition to fat and lactose, dairy contains components such as whey and casein, which can cause severe digestion problems.*

**Egg yolks** (whites are fine, do try to buy organic)

Meat, dairy products, and egg yolks are particularly dangerous for all aspects of IBS. In some people their high fat content causes violent, rapid colon spasms and triggers diarrhea. Alternately, for others their heavy animal proteins, complete lack of fiber, and very low water content can lead to drastically slowed colon contractions and severe constipation. No matter what IBS symptoms you're prone to, these three foods pose high risks and are really best eliminated from your diet altogether.

| | |
|---|---|
| **French fries** | **Corn dogs** |
| **Onion rings** | ***Anything* battered and deep-** |
| **Fried chicken** | **fried** |

*Anything* skillet-fried in fat of
any kind

Shortening

Margarine

All oils, fats, spreads, etc.

Mayonnaise

Salad dressings

Tartar sauce

Cool Whip

Coconut milk

Shredded coconut

Solid chocolate (baking
cocoa powder is fine)

Solid carob (carob powder is
fine)

Olives

Nuts and nut butters

Croissants, pastries, biscuits,
scones, and doughnuts

Pie crust

Potato chips (unless they're
baked)

Corn chips and nachos
(unless they're baked)

Dried bananas (they're
almost always deep fried)

---

[19] Please don't fall for the conclusively disproven belief that dairy products are necessary for calcium and thus strong bones, and that milk reduces the risk of osteoporosis. Reams of studies over decades have shown no benefits whatsoever to dairy calcium regarding bone loss. The sulfate released from animal protein amino acid loads (in both dairy and meat) causes an over-acid condition in your body, due to the formation of uric acid and metabolic wastes. To remedy this situation your body must leach alkaline minerals, namely calcium and magnesium, out of your bones to buffer the acid, and these minerals are then excreted through urine. As a result, each time you eat dairy products (or meat) your body actually suffers a net calcium loss. [Breslau, N. "Relationship of Animal Protein-rich Diet to Kidney Stone Formation and Calcium Metabolism." *J Clin Endocrinol Metab* 66 (1988): 140.] The Harvard Nurses' Health Study (Feskanich D., et al., "Milk, Dietary Calcium, and Bone Fractures in Women: A Twelve-Year Prospective Study," *Am J Public Health* 87 (1997): 992–997] which followed more than seventy-five thousand women for twelve years, showed no protective effect of increased milk consumption on fracture risk. In fact, increased intake of calcium from dairy products was associated with a *higher* fracture risk. An Australian study [Cumming R.G., and R.J. Klineberg, "Case-control Study of Risk Factors for Hip Fractures in the Elderly," *Am J Epidem* 139 (1994): 493–505] showed the same results. Additionally, other studies [Huang Z., J.H. Himes, and P.G. McGovern, "Nutrition and Subsequent Hip Fracture Risk among a National Cohort of White Women," *Am J Epidem* 144: 124–34, and Cummings, S.R., et al., "Risk Factors for Hip Fracture in White Women," *N Engl J Med* 332 (1996): 767–773] have also found no protective effect of dairy calcium on bone. You can decrease your risk of osteoporosis by reducing sodium and animal protein intake in the diet, increasing intake of fruits and vegetables, exercising, and ensuring adequate calcium intake from plant foods such as leafy green vegetables and beans, as well as calcium-fortified products such as breakfast cereals and juices. See also *Eating for IBS*, by Heather Van Vorous (Marlowe & Company, 2000).

allows me to prevent problems from snack to snack and meal to meal, but in the end it adds up to long-term stability from day to day, week to week, and even month to month. I've never found a better method for completely preventing my IBS symptoms than basing my diet on soluble fiber foods.

You can keep your colon stabilized each and every day by basing all meals and snacks on soluble fiber foods.

## Fat—The bad guy

Well, you probably knew this one. Most people quickly figure out on their own that greasy foods cause problems. High-fat foods are usually easy to identify, and after getting sick for the third or fourth time in a row after eating French fries or ice cream it becomes painfully obvious that fat is an IBS trigger. Have you been wondering why?

Fat is the single greatest digestive tract stimulant. Nothing else will trigger a more powerful gastrocolic reflex. For those of us already prone to wildly unstable colon contractions, this is bad news indeed. Interestingly, the type of fat doesn't matter at all—saturated, monounsaturated, polyunsaturated, they're all equal triggers. It simply makes no difference to your gastrocolic reflex if you're eating lard or imported-from-a-village-in-Tuscany extra-virgin olive oil. It will make quite a difference to your heart and your health in general, of course, but in terms of controlling IBS the less fat of all kinds, the better—period. This doesn't mean following a fat-free diet, by the way, but simply a low-fat one.

Fats are usually fairly obvious foods to identify, but not always. The worst culprits are listed in the side bar, and many (particularly meat, dairy, egg yolks, and fried foods) can simply be eliminated from your diet entirely and your whole body will be healthier for it.

I know the thought of this can be deeply shocking, but giving up these foods does *not* equal deprivation. Honestly, it doesn't—I promise. There are a great many easy substitutions that will let you cook and eat safely while still enjoying many of your traditional favorite foods. There's also a lot of fun to be had in trying a wide variety of new ones. And when you're tempted to indulge in a dangerous treat, just remember that everything tastes a lot less delicious when it's followed by a vicious IBS attack.

There are also some hidden sources of fat to watch out for. Cookies, crackers, pancakes, waffles, French toast, biscuits, scones, pastries, dough-nuts, and mashed potatoes can all be sky-high in fat (virtually always so at restaurants), so be careful. Give thanks for the recent fat-free craze that has given us supermarket aisles full of safe alternatives. I certainly would have killed for fat-free Saltines as a kid. Every time I had an attack I was given soda crackers—and I sure wish I'd known then why this so often made me worse, not better.

## Insoluble fiber—good or bad?

Both! Here's the type of fiber everyone is familiar with—bran, whole grains, raw fruits and vegetables (note the exceptions under Soluble Fiber), greens, sprouts, legumes, seeds, and nuts. In short, the healthi-est foods in the world, and what everyone should be eating as much of as possible. Right? Well, right, except for one small problem. Insoluble fiber, like fat, is a very powerful GI tract stimulant, and for those of us with IBS this can spell big trouble. Unlike fat, however, you cannot sim-ply minimize your insoluble fiber intake, as this will leave you with a seriously unhealthy diet. It's a catch-22, but the conflict can be solved fairly easily.

## Insoluble Fiber Foods—Eat with Care

**ONE GLANCE** will tell you these are the best (and tastiest) foods around, but your colon simply can't handle it if you eat them with abandon. You can (and absolutely *must*) eat them, but within the IBS dietary guidelines. Treat these foods with suitable caution, and you'll be able to enjoy a wide variety of them, in very healthy quantities, without problem.

In general, if a plant food (no animal products contain fiber) seems rough, stringy, has a tough skin, hull, peel, pod, or seeds, be careful. This is not a comprehensive list by any means but it should give you the general idea.

Whole wheat flour, whole wheat bread, whole wheat cereal

Bran

Whole grains, whole grain breads, whole grain cereals

Granola

Meusli

Seeds

Nuts

Popcorn

Beans and lentils (mashed or puréed they're much safer)

Berries (blueberries, strawberries, blackberries, cranberries, etc.)

Grapes and raisins

Cherries

Pineapple

Peaches, nectarines, apricots, and pears with skins (peeled they're much safer)

Apples (peeled they're safe)

Rhubarb

Melons

Oranges, grapefruits, lemons, limes

Dates and prunes

Greens (spinach, lettuce, kale, mesclun, collards, arugala, watercress, etc.)

Whole peas, snow peas, snap peas, pea pods

Green beans

Kernel corn

Bell peppers (roasted and peeled they're safer)

Eggplant (peeled and seeded it's much safer)

Celery

Onions, shallots, leeks, scallions, garlic

Cabbage, bok choy, Brussels sprouts

Broccoli

Cauliflower

Tomatoes (peeled and seeded, especially raw, they're much safer)

Cucumbers (again, peel and seed them and they're much safer)

**Sprouts** (alfalfa, sunflower, radish, etc.)

Fresh herbs

*Never eat insoluble fiber alone or on an empty stomach. Always eat it with a larger quantity of soluble fiber, and you will keep your gastrocolic reflex stable.* What does this mean in practical terms? Cook some diced vegetables into a low-fat sauce for pasta, stir-fry veggies into a fried rice, or blend fresh fruit into a smoothie to drink after a breakfast bowl of oatmeal. *For fruits, vegetables, and legumes in general, peeling, chopping, cooking, and puréeing them will significantly minimize the impact of their insoluble fiber.*

Make soups, drinks, sauces, breads, and dips from your veggies and fruits instead of eating them whole and raw. For beans and lentils, cook and blend them into sauces, dips, soups, or spreads—their insoluble fiber is found in their outer skins and their insides are actually rich in soluble fiber. For nuts, finely grind and incorporate them into breads or cakes with white flour, which gives a safe soluble fiber base. For bran and other whole grains, eat them in small quantities following soluble fiber foods— have a little whole wheat dinner roll after a big sourdough one, or mix a small amount of fat-free granola into a large bowl of cream of rice or Corn Chex cereal. For raw fruit and green salads, eat them at the end of a soluble fiber meal instead of at the beginning. For all insoluble fiber foods, start with small quantities and gradually increase your intake, making sure you follow the guidelines in the upcoming Day 3 Living section.

Some fruits and vegetables are particularly troublesome for IBS:

**Sulfur-containing foods** (garlic, onions, leeks, broccoli, cauliflower, cabbage, asparagus, and Brussels sprouts), in addition to their high amounts of insoluble fiber, also produce significant gas in the GI tract and this can trigger attacks. As with all other fruits and veggies, however, these are extremely nutritious foods with significant health benefits, so they need to be treated with caution but definitely not eliminated from your diet.

**Acidic foods** (citrus fruits and cooked tomatoes) should be treated with extra care as well, as their acidity can cause both upper and lower GI distress. Once again, follow the rules for insoluble fiber and eat these foods in smaller quantities incorporated with soluble fiber—but please do eat them.

**Fructose,** a fruit sugar, can cause gas, bloating, and diarrhea (this is typically not true for sucrose, or plain table sugar). Fruit juices, particularly apple and grape juice, are often sky-high in fructose and even more problematic than whole fresh fruit. It's simply much easier and faster to drink a large glass of juice (and ingest a great deal of fructose)

# I'm Confused! How Can the Same Food Have Insoluble and Soluble Fiber?

**MOST ALL** grains, cereals, legumes, and tubers have an outer insoluble fiber layer, and a soluble fiber interior (and the same is true for some fruits and vegetables, such as apples and zucchini). It's very easy to actually see this with your own eyes. If you take a cooked grain of brown rice, wheat berry, kernel of corn, potato, or bean you can separate the tough exterior (the bran, skin, or shell) from the creamy interior. When the bran is removed from wheat berries and they're milled the result is white flour; when the bran is removed from brown rice the result is white rice. There aren't many similar common commercial processes that remove the insoluble fiber exterior from legumes, fruits, or vegetables, but finely blending, puréeing, or peeling these whole foods will greatly minimize their trigger risk.

Wheat in particular causes confusion for many, many people with IBS who are unsure about whether or not it is a safe food for them. There is no flat "yes" or "no" answer to this concern because, as we've just learned, it depends. Whole wheat, with its outer layer of bran, is high in insoluble fiber. This means that it's a trigger. That's why whole wheat bread, whole wheat cereals, and bran can cause such awful problems for people with IBS. [20]

However, when you remove the bran from whole wheat you end up with white flour (the regular kind you can buy in any grocery store, that you using in baking breads, muffins, etc.). Though this is still wheat flour, it is not *whole wheat* flour, and this makes a world of difference. White flour contains no insoluble fiber but it does have soluble fiber, which is the stabilizing force of the IBS diet (just picture the thick gel that results when you dissolve a piece of white bread in a glass of water). This is why white breads are such great safe staples.

When you read the ingredients on packaged foods they might not specify if the wheat flour used is "white" or "whole," but it's usually pretty easy to tell. For breads, a brief glance will tell you if there is whole wheat in it (you'll see little brown flakes). If the bread is pure white, like French or sourdough, you're safe. For most crackers, pretzels, muffins, and so on, only white flour will be used. The exception is health food store products, which are likely to use whole wheat. However, they will almost always tout this fact so you won't be left wondering.

---

[20] Francis C. Y. and P. J. Whorwell. "Bran and the Irritable Bowel Syndrome: Time for Reappraisal." *Lancet* 344 (1994): 19–24.

The whole wheat (and other insoluble fiber) intolerances so common to IBS are markedly different from true food allergies. If you're allergic to wheat, it will make no difference if the grain is left whole or refined by removing the bran. In addition, with many allergies even minuscule quantities of the trigger, whether eaten with other foods or alone, can trigger violent reactions. Fortunately, with IBS this is rarely the case, so we just have to be careful with whole wheat and other insoluble fibers. If we do take care we can easily and frequently eat them in small quantities when they're combined with high soluble fiber foods. In addition, with wheat, once the bran has been removed so has the risk of an IBS attack, and this gives us great dietary freedom when it comes to white breads and other refined wheat flour foods.

than to eat an equivalent amount of whole fruit. So treat juices as you would insoluble fiber and drink them carefully, with soluble fiber foods.

## Other pesky creatures to avoid

Coffee—both regular and decaf—contains an enzyme that's an extremely powerful GI tract irritant. Go cold turkey today and drink herbal teas instead. **Caffeine** is a GI stimulant and should be avoided, especially in higher doses. **Alcohol** is a GI irritant and often triggers attacks, especially on an empty stomach (though small amounts of alcohol used in cooking are fine). **Carbonation** in soda pop and mineral water can cause bloating and cramps. **Artificial sweeteners**, particularly sorbitol, can trigger pain and diarrhea. Artificial fats, namely **Olestra**, can cause abdominal cramping and diarrhea in people who don't even have IBS—imagine what it can do to you. **MSG** has acquired lots of ugly anecdotal evidence against it regarding all sorts of digestive upsets. It can simply be avoided, so why take a chance?

## Size matters

No matter how safe any food is for IBS, eating a huge portion of it in one sitting can trigger an attack. Your gastrocolic reflex gains strength in direct correlation to the number of calories you consume in a meal. While this makes it easy to see why high fat foods cause problems (fat is more than twice as calorie-dense as carbohydrates and proteins), it also means that bingeing—on anything—carries serious risks for those of us with IBS. So don't kid yourself that when your friends break out a pint of Chunky Monkey and a spoon for that video you're watching, you can do the same with fat-free sorbet. It's not just ingredients, but quantity too. Size really does matter.

Keeping your portions small has some fringe benefits, particularly in that it should make it easier to eat more frequently, and this is a helpful strategy for maintaining a constant intake of soluble fiber. Unfortunately, Americans have gotten used to "super-sizing" just about everything they eat, and this can be a hard habit to break. One thing to try at home is serving yourself on salad plates and soup bowls, so that visually you don't feel faced with a skimpy meal. Remember too that you can always take a second small portion after you finish the first one, as long as you eat at a slow-to-moderate pace and you still feel hungry. This is a great way to keep from over-serving yourself initially and then feeling obligated to eat everything on your plate even if you're full (a "don't waste food" lesson ingrained in most of us as children).

Snacking on small amounts of food throughout the day will keep you from getting ravenous and then overeating, which can trigger an attack. At restaurants (which are covered thoroughly in Week 3) make a point of dividing your plate in half the moment you're served and take that portion home with you for a later meal. Once you develop this habit you'll likely be astonished to realize how oversized most restaurant meals are, and it will be clear why it's so common to suffer an attack if you eat all that food at one sitting. I have a few favorite restaurants (Ethiopian and Middle Eastern) whose dinner portions are so generous I actually get three complete meals out of them. Even someone without IBS is likely to feel pretty uncomfortable if they down that much food at one dinner.

# Will Eating for IBS Make Me Fat?

**YOU'RE NOT** alone if you're wondering whether eating safely for IBS will lead to excess weight gain. Rest assured, it won't. The basis of the IBS diet, soluble fiber, has no calories at all as it is indigestible. High soluble fiber foods are virtually always high in complex carbohydrates and low in fat. This is a good thing, as the healthiest diets in the world, associated with the lowest obesity rates, are those highest in complex carbohydrates and lowest in fat and protein (particularly from animal products). This fact completely contradicts the current and misguided popularity of high protein/low carbohydrate fad diets. Tellingly, the obesity rates for cultures with high carb/low fat and protein diets (primarily in Asia) are a fraction of the obesity rates in the U.S. We average only 40–50% of diet from carbohydrates–but most Asian nations average 60–75%. Our national obesity rate is now one of the highest in the *world,* at 35% for adults and 20% for children.[21] The average Asian country's obesity rate is just 2–3%.[22] Striking, isn't it? On a personal note, I have eaten the IBS diet since late childhood (I'm now in my early thirties) and have never weighed over one hundred twenty pounds at 5'6." I don't count calories or restrict what I eat aside from IBS triggers, I am not an exercise fanatic, and I'm not somehow genetically gifted with a skinny gene. It has simply never been possible to eat enough high soluble fiber foods (they're very filling) to gain weight while still keeping my diet low fat.

The high soluble fiber diet necessary for controlling IBS should actually result in weight loss–*if* you're overweight.[23] If your weight is already normal it won't result in weight gain unless you significantly up your portion sizes, which would likely trigger an attack, or gorge yourself on refined sugar foods that have no soluble fiber to fill you up. The IBS diet is essentially low-fat vegetarian-based, plus chicken breasts and seafood.Eliminating the meat, dairy, fried foods, and soda pop drastically lowers the calorie count for people who switch from a "typical" American diet. Upping your soluble fiber food intake will increase your calories from complex carbohydrates, but these are much less calorie-dense

---

[21] The National Center for Health Statistics, and Federal Centers for Disease Control and Prevention.
[22] World Health Organization, 1998.

than all the fats you've eliminated. It also takes more energy for your body to store excess carbohydrates, versus excess fats, as body fat, so you have to eat more carbohydrate calories than fat calories in order to gain weight.

Carefully incorporating as much insoluble fiber as you can tolerate will not add any significant calories at all. Plus, both types of fiber are very filling, and will help with appetite control. Eating small portions frequently, important for minimizing the risk of attacks, also helps keep you filled without having to eat as much.

Finally, please realize that soluble fiber is extremely beneficial for a lot of health problems besides IBS. It not only regulates and normalizes colonic activity, it also lowers LDL ("bad" blood cholesterol levels and the corresponding risk of heart disease, prevents colon cancer, and improves glycemic (blood sugar) control in diabetics by slowing the digestion of carbohydrates and subsequent release of glucose into the blood. It also helps prevent blood vessel constriction and the formation of free radicals—both risk factors for heart attacks—by slowing the absorption of fat and carbohydrates into the bloodstream.[24] Best of all, it really and truly does dramatically help prevent IBS attacks. So don't be afraid of it, and don't worry about weight gain or difficult weight loss. Eating for IBS should safely and easily normalize your weight, helping you lose pounds if you need to. And if you're looking for a weight gain, finally having the knowledge of how to eat without fear should allow you to up your calorie intake significantly and add on the pounds you need for good health.

---

[23] Following the publication of *Eating for IBS* I received many letters from people as thrilled with their incidental weight loss (anywhere from thirty-five to eighty pounds) from the diet as with the elimination of their IBS symptoms. Some had actually had friends and family members begin following the IBS diet solely because they were overweight.

[24] Dr. David L. Katz, Yale School of Medicine, New Haven, Connecticut, presenting findings at the 1999 meeting of the American College of Nutrition, held in Washington, D.C.

There's another aspect to portion control that has some happy possibilities for IBS. The risk of trigger foods can be tremendously minimized if they're eaten in tiny quantities following soluble fiber. In this regard, it is as much *how* you eat as *what* you eat that will help you manage your symptoms. While this is most important as a tool to allow you to incorporate all those healthy insoluble fiber foods as often as possible, it's also a means of treating yourself to a "mini-splurge" every once in a while. Let's say you're well-stabilized and just dying for a Snickers. Eating a full-size candy bar as a snack when your stomach is empty will likely wreak havoc and send you into an immediate downward spiral of attacks (why? because it's sky-high in fat and dairy, and very little soluble fiber).

However, if your symptoms were well under control and you instead decided to treat yourself to a snack-size individual Snickers bar (a tiny portion equals a tiny quantity of fat/dairy triggers) for dessert, immediately following a nice low-fat, high soluble fiber meal, you'd likely do just fine. I eat solid chocolate almost every day in this manner. (Of course, this may just be sheer willpower because as God is my witness I will not go through life without chocolate, but I think this is probably the less likely explanation.)

Whatever your favorite trigger food, this strategy gives you a good means of allowing yourself the occasional small indulgence. IBS food intolerances are, fortunately, not like food allergies, where the quantity of a trigger (say, peanuts) may not matter. For this we can thank our lucky stars, as it means that few things are truly forbidden to us as long as we follow some common sense rules and exercise a little self control. Now, where's that Hershey's Kiss I've been saving?

*living*

# The Ten Commandments of Eating for IBS

**IS YOUR** head spinning from all these new categories of food? Don't worry. I know it can be confusing at first to start thinking about what you eat in terms of fats and types of fibers. But what seems foreign today will be old hat tomorrow, so just take things one day at a time. Making the effort here is truly worthwhile, because following the IBS diet will make a world of difference in your life.

Feeling skeptical? Wondering just how much of an improvement the IBS diet can really make? Well, for me eating properly means the difference between being desperately, violently ill every single day of my life and suffering an attack out of the blue a few times a year. That fits my definition of overwhelming success, and fortunately I'm not alone here. Similar—and even better—results have been reached by literally thousands of other IBS sufferers who have written me to say so.

*"I cannot tell you what following Heather's IBS dietary
information has done for me.
I am now a normal person."*

—KIT GORRELL, Overland Park, Kansas,
IBS Sufferer for 6 years.

*"Crisis knocked on my door in 1995—three times. In March I lost
my job and my marriage, within two weeks of each other. In July I lost
my brother to cancer. And then my body's 'absorption' of crisis took the
form of IBS. One never gives digestion a second thought, it seems, until
it doesn't work properly. In the summer of 1995 my digestive system
suddenly revolted, and everything that once was normal and 'daily'
became very different, and 'ten times per day.' We often laugh at the TV
commercial of the poor man sitting in the inside seat of the crowded
airplane, who has been hit with diarrhea and is hurriedly trying to
make his way to the back of the plane to the bathroom; but unless you
have been in this situation, day in and day out, you cannot know the
anguish, the fear, the anxiety that this situation brings upon you. It is
anything but humorous. It is enough to make you give up all trips and
vacations, to never venture too far from home, and on bad days, to
never leave the house at all. IBS makes you question your choices of
clothing, friends, and your job. It deprives you of peace of mind, of freedom, of being a normal person in every sense of the word. It makes one
live in fear. It can deeply affect your relationships, including those with
ones you hold most dear. It can affect every facet of your life. My life
became just like this.*

*I spent two years thinking that 'it will just go away' when I've had
time to emotionally heal. After two years I found myself at my doctor's,
discussing other issues, and I happened to bring up the fact that I had
had diarrhea continually for two years. My doctor stated that 'this is
just your body's new normal due to the stress in your life. Don't worry
about it.' I was stupid. I believed this completely idiotic statement, and
continued on my path of daily hell. I waited another year and a half,
and saw another doctor, again for an unrelated problem. Again I mentioned the diarrhea, and this doctor said, 'This is not normal, not at all.
I'm referring you to a specialist. You need a colonoscopy immediately.'
Within a week I had had the procedure done, was prescribed a med-*

ication, and promptly released with no further contact from my doctor. There was never any discussion of my dietary habits, and what I might be unknowingly doing to cause my system to be in such a state. I was left to fight the battle on my own.

After another year of no improvement, I went back to the specialist, and was given a new anti-diarrhea medication. Still, nothing worked. Not only did the medications have no effect, but things were now getting worse. I was unable to make the twenty-minute drive to work without stopping at least twice to go to the bathroom. I was unable to attend a conference two hours away from work because I knew it was a possibly disastrous situation. Then I had to take a trip to St. Louis, and found myself early in the morning, in a shuttle van going to the airport, stopping at various hotels along the way to pick up passengers. By the time I arrived at the airport, I was clutching my friend's hand, in tears, and truly pale from trying to hold back on my body's natural morning tendencies. She was a wonderful friend who knew of my situation, and reassured me that whatever happened, it would be OK. We could handle it together. While literally running to the bathroom after being let off the shuttle, I realized that I could no longer live this way. When I returned home, I would find an answer; I would become a normal person again if it was the last thing I did.

The very next day, I found the book Eating for IBS and was thrown a lifeline, and given the information to find my life again, to find sanity, peace of mind, and to feel better than I have in a very long time. I thought I had nowhere to turn, and no one to ask for help, but here was my answer. I read the information and first balked at all the things that I loved that I would have to 'give up': coffee (my number one dietary pleasure), red meat, dairy products, fats, caffeine, etc. But I realized that I was staring my salvation in the face, and to feel better, to become a normal person in every sense of the word, was worth anything I might give up in my diet. I was at the point that I would do whatever it took. I read the information maybe ten times to fully understand what I was doing. In addition, I e-mailed the author, fully sure that I would never hear a reply from someone who had written a book on the subject. I was shocked…not only did I get a response, but it was within hours! Heather promised that I would feel better in a matter of days, and that within two weeks my life would be on its way back to being normal. She was absolutely right. I followed every suggestion she offered. I gladly threw my coffee away, moved the drip coffee maker to the basement, stocked up on peppermint tea, Metamucil, rice, and everything else recommended.

My diarrhea, which had sent me in search of the bathroom ten to fourteen times per day, within two days was down to once or twice. I continued the diet, feeling relief for the first time in over five years. By two weeks, my stool had regained its normalcy, and I remember crying the first time I had a normal bowel movement. It was certainly cause for a private celebration. Unless you are in this situation, this might sound humorous, or even ridiculous. But if you have IBS, you know exactly what I'm talking about.

I have been on the IBS diet since October 2000. After giving myself a full month of strict adherence to the diet, I began to introduce some favorites back into my eating, to see what the results might be. I have never brought drip coffee (caffeinated or decaf) back into my diet, as I feel this was the major contribution of my IBS. I have learned to love herbal teas, and peppermint tea is one of the simplest, most basic and powerful contributions to this diet. I am now able to successfully tolerate Folgers Decaf coffee in tea bag form. Since I love coffee, this was a great find for me! I continue to make soluble fiber the basis and foundation of my diet. I eat a great deal of bananas and rice. I omit beef almost entirely from my diet, as well as pork. I rarely have pop, and when I do, it is always 7-Up or Sprite, never anything with caffeine or the diet varieties. I find that when I go out to eat, and have a heavy meal of foods higher in fat, it causes problems and my IBS can flare almost immediately. Eating simply what is recommended yields the best results. I have learned to live without pepperoni pizza, drip coffee, a good juicy steak, and many other foods that I love. It simply is not worth returning to my former life.

A side benefit is that I began losing weight from my dietary changes. I began exercising, and at present I have dropped four clothing sizes, going from a size sixteen to a size eight. Exercise certainly has helped, but the change in my diet has had a tremendous impact.

I cannot tell you what finding Heather's IBS dietary information has done for me. I am now a normal person. My day is no longer regulated by where the bathroom is, how long it might take for me to find it *or get to it, or giving up normal aspects of life such as travel and going out to eat on a date. I am infuriated that the medical community would rather prescribe medication than address the logical impact that diet has upon digestion. I have been off all medication I had taken for IBS since October 2000. I do not envision having to go back to my gastroenterologist in the future. And when crisis comes and knocks on my door now, I am healthier and better able to send it on its way without lasting repercussions."*

I hope you're feeling inspired. Now that you've got the information, and you've got the guidelines, all you need is a game plan. Let's take the knowledge of how to eat safely and put it into practical terms.

## The ten commandments of eating for IBS

1. *Always* eat soluble fiber first, eat soluble fiber whenever your stomach is empty, and make soluble fiber foods the largest component of every meal and snack.
2. Minimize your fat intake to twenty-five percent of your diet, *max*. Read labels and, at restaurants, ask.
3. Never eat high-fat foods, even in small portions, on an empty stomach or without soluble fiber. Better still, don't eat them at all.
4. Eliminate all red meat, dairy, fried foods, egg yolks, coffee, soda pop, and alcohol from your diet. This may be the most difficult dietary strategy to adopt, and I know it probably won't be fun or easy—but neither are IBS attacks.
5. Never, never, never eat insoluble fiber on an empty stomach, in large quantities at one sitting, or without soluble fiber.
6. Eat small portions frequently, calmly, and leisurely.
7. If you're unsure about something, *don't eat it*. It's not worth the risk.
8. Food is fun and eating should be pleasurable. Take the time and make the effort to eat safely, and then enjoy yourself.
9. Remember that you have *absolute* and *total* control over your diet. No one can force you to eat something you know you shouldn't— if anyone tries, think of them as a drug dealer and just say no.
10. Practice creative substitution, not deprivation. Use soy or rice replacements for dairy, two egg whites to replace a whole egg, try

low-fat vegetarian versions of meat products, replace some oil with fruit puréees in breads or cakes, use veggie broth instead of oil in sauces, bake with cocoa powder (it's very low fat) instead of solid chocolate. Use herbs, baking extracts (vanilla, peppermint, maple, etc.), and mild spices generously to heighten flavors.

If you're currently trying to break the cycle of ongoing attacks, it is best to strictly limit your diet to soluble fiber foods and peppermint tea for several days. This will allow your GI tract to stabilize, and then you can gradually and carefully add in other foods following the rules. At that point you'll be ready to go shopping, restock the pantry with your new safe staples, and learn how to cook fast, easy, fabulous meals following the IBS guidelines.

## IN A SENTENCE:

*Learning the dietary categories of soluble fiber, fat, and insoluble fiber is the key to understanding how foods can help or hurt IBS.*

# DAY **4**

*task list*

> 1. **BEGIN (OR MAINTAIN) A DAILY, ENJOYABLE EXERCISE ROUTINE, WHETHER AT OR OUTSIDE OF YOUR HOME.**

# Keep Active to Stay Healthy

**EXERCISE, IN** any way, shape, form, duration, and intensity that appeals to you, will help you deal with IBS more successfully both physically and mentally. All that really matters here is that you do it and you enjoy it.

It's not just a hopeful theory that staying active will significantly improve your physical and mental health. The research findings on the subject are overwhelming at this point. Study after study proves that exercise increases longevity and decreases mortality from a wide range of diseases.[25] In fact,

---

[25] The specific health benefits of exercise include: greater longevity; improved cardiovascular health; lower risks of diabetes, arthritis, osteoporosis, cancer, lung disease, gastrointestinal disorders; common colds and flu, and leg cramps; improvements to central nervous system diseases; healthier pregnancies; prevention and cure of obesity; and promotion of psychological and emotional well-being including mental acuity, reaction time, creativity, and imagination. (*What Are the Specific Benefits of Exercise?*

inactivity should be considered a diseased state, given that exercise is absolutely known to:

- ○ Reduce muscle tension. Exercise works your muscles, releasing the energy they've stored from involuntary contractions under stress, and allows them to relax. When your muscles are relaxed you will be too—and so will your colon.
- ○ Increase your ability to fight illness. When you're physically fit it's not just muscles that function better, but internal organs as well. This includes the organs of your digestive tract. The greater physical stamina and resiliency you'll gain from exercise will not only reduce your risk of suffering an IBS attack in the first place, but allow you to more quickly recover from one.
- ○ Regulate bowel function and increase the efficiency of your entire digestive process. In particular, few things are more effective than exercise for preventing and relieving constipation.
- ○ Provide a healthy catharsis for stressful emotions such as anger and hostility, allowing their productive, physical dissipation. Tomorrow you'll learn just how sensitive the colons of IBS sufferers are to negative emotions, and why it's crucial that you release these feelings. Exercise is an ideal way.

Exercise is also a great way to:

- ○ Produce endorphins, brain chemicals that act as painkillers and can induce a state of euphoria. Exercise is in fact so beneficial to creating a positive mood that it is considered an effective treatment for clinical depression. Imagine what it will do for you when you're just having a bum day.
- ○ Improve the quality of your sleep. One of the first signs of stress is the frustration of tossing and turning all night long, and you'll learn on Day 5 just how a sleepless night directly corresponds to an IBS morning. Exercise leads to a healthy, pleasant exhaustion that allows you to fall asleep more easily and then sleep more soundly.

---

Well-Connected via WebMD.com, Harvey Simon, M.D., Editor-in-Chief, Nidus Information Services, Inc., 41 East 11th Street, 11th Floor, New York.)

○ Reduce the biochemical impact of worry and stress on your body. When you're under stress, neurotransmitters are activated, hormones released, cortisol produced, and entire body systems accelerate or slow their functions. IBS attack, anyone? The by-products of this response can continue to negatively impact your body and health. Exercise minimizes the effect of these by-products and reduces their physical impact.

○ Provide a form of moving meditation. Any exercise that involves a consistent repetitive motion can alter your state of consciousness. In other words, you'll obtain the beneficial effects of meditation (which are dealt with directly in tomorrow's chapter) without actually meditating. Your breathing and movement during exercise can produce a state of tranquility and calmness in the aftermath, giving you pronounced physiological benefits.

○ Improve your self-image and increase your self-esteem, both of which directly correlate to a greater ability to tolerate stress. People who exercise feel better about themselves, are less susceptible to stress, and thus less prone to IBS attacks.

○ Allow both introspective solitude and social support. Depending on your personal preference and choice of sport, exercise can provide you with a solitary escape from stress (long runs down quiet country roads) or a recreational play period with teammates who share the fun (softball games in the park). Both offer a respite from daily worries, an increase in energy levels, and reduced levels of stress. Choose one form of activity or the other, or alternate between the two. Either way you win and your IBS loses.

*living*

# Get Your Exercise

*"I know from experience that after I exercise
I will definitely feel better."*

—MINDY HELM, 22 years old, Kent, Washington,
IBS sufferer for 3 years.

*"I was always a very active person who exercised every day
until I first developed IBS three years ago. As I became
sicker and sicker, my energy level dropped to a very low
point and I eventually had to quit exercising altogether
because I just didn't have the strength. At this point (it had
been a whole year) I finally saw a doctor and was diagnosed
with both IBS and lactose intolerance. I felt like I'd been
hit by a truck when I heard the news. Although I then tried
to stay away from dairy (my favorite foods), this didn't really help me that much. Eating more soluble fiber did help,
but I still didn't feel great. I decided to slowly start working
out again, and I eventually increased my workouts to the
most strenuous, frequent level possible. Although it didn't
happen overnight, my symptoms did gradually decrease
and one day I realized that I once again felt good.*

*The whole experience of IBS has been very frustrating to me. Ironically, exercise has helped me as much with this frustration as with the IBS itself, particularly my dismay over not being able to eat whatever I want, whenever I want. Exercise also helps me manage my daily stress levels, and for me stress is a huge trigger. Today, even when my IBS is acting up and I'm not feeling so great, I'll go for a run in spite of it all. Invariably, I'll feel so much better when my workout's through. It's still hard for me to remain motivated on the days I'm not doing well, but now I know from experience that after I exercise, in any way at all, I will definitely feel better. For me, exercise is **always** worth my time."*

If you already have a regular workout routine you're surely well aware of the benefits to your entire life and health, and IBS just adds another motivating factor for sticking with your physical activities. However, if you're faced with starting a new exercise program, this is a little more difficult than merely staying with one that's well-established and that you enjoy. It helps a lot to mentally take just one step at a time here, and make it your goal to be physically active *today*. Consider yourself a person in exercise recovery, and don't worry about tomorrow until you get there. Trying to begin a routine with the outlook that this is a lifelong venture is likely to seem overwhelming, if not completely insurmountable. This mindset will just set you up for failure and depression. Instead, take the small step of exercising today, tonight, or first thing tomorrow morning, and make sure to mentally congratulate yourself when you finish. Start each day fresh, so yesterday's missed workout is irrelevant today.

If it's been awhile since you were physically active, you may have to fight the urge you're likely to feel to just stay home today and start your workouts tomorrow...but tomorrow never comes. You may not feel like learning a new sport, taking a class, changing for the gym, or bothering with lessons. If this is the case, stop worrying about it, and simply go outside and walk. Or get inside on a treadmill and walk. Or go to your local mall and walk (don't shop, just walk). Do this today, tomorrow, and every day after that, and your entire body and state of health, as well as your IBS symptoms, are bound to be the better for it.

If you do have the energy and feel excited about taking a bigger step and joining in a true sport, but are at a loss as to where to begin, it may help to think back to your favorite activity in grade school, high school, or college. Did you love basketball? tennis? swimming? dancing? Whatever it was, remember how much you enjoyed it at the time, and try to find a way to get the sport back into your life. Most of us enjoyed playing games and running, skipping, jumping our way through childhood, but lost this element of sheer physical joy from our daily lives as we got older. This is what exercise can bring back into your adult life, not just good physical and mental health. You do have to make an effort, but the rewards are truly worthwhile.

It's helpful to remember that exercise is not a quick fix that will immediately halt all IBS symptoms, but rather something you need to devote time to, preferably every single day, for the rest of your life. Just as IBS is an ongoing syndrome so physical activity, like diet, is an ongoing solution. The results from exercise will only equal your dedication, so make it a priority. Your health deserves it.

## Resources

Your local gym—just check the yellow pages under "health clubs"
YMCA/YWCA
Local league sports
Company or corporate teams
School sports for students
Exercise videotapes
Home exercise equipment
A comfy pair of sneakers and the world outside your door

## IN A SENTENCE:

> *Exercise of any kind can be crucial to helping you successfully deal with IBS both physically and mentally, so find an enjoyable way to keep active and stick with it.*

DAY**5**

*learning*

*task list*

1. MAKE A COMMITMENT TO YOURSELF TO
   GET ENOUGH SLEEP EACH NIGHT, OR A
   NAP EACH DAY.

2. BEGIN A DAILY FORM OF STRESS
   MANAGEMENT: THERAPEUTIC HEAT,
   MEDITATION, YOGA, TAI CHI, OR ANY
   OTHER PREFERRED PRACTICE THAT
   INDUCES RELAXATION AND
   INTROSPECTION.

# Stress—
# How to Wrestle It
# into Submission

**THE POTENTIAL** for abnormal colon function is always
present in people with IBS, but a trigger must be present to
actually cause symptoms. Along with diet, stress is the greatest trigger there is.

Stress inhibits the sympathetic nerve plexuses, and stimulates excessive adrenaline production, which in turn upsets
the rhythmic muscle contractions of the gut. Given that people with IBS are prone to suffer from irregular GI contractions

by definition, it's easy to see why stress is such a powerful trigger. Several interesting studies have actually shown the direct link between emotional stressors and subsequent IBS flares.

One experiment with eighteen IBS patients investigated how different emotions would affect the muscle contractions of the colon. The patients were hypnotized and instructed to feel anger, excitement, or happiness. Colonic motility rates were measured, and found to increase significantly with anger and excitement. Happiness reduced colonic spasms, although interestingly, the hypnosis itself had already had this effect to a lesser degree (more on hypnotherapy as a treatment for IBS on Day 7).[26] A second study specifically looked at the effect of anger on the colon. Even at rest, patients with IBS had more active colons than the control subjects, and they demonstrated significantly greater colon muscle contractions than the controls when angered.[27] Yet another recent study has confirmed a direct relationship between daily stress and the level of IBS symptoms, finding a significant and positive correlation between the two.[28]

However, I'm guessing you're already well aware of these facts, thanks to plenty of painful personal experience. The question now is, what can you do about it? First, be aware of what actually causes stress in your daily life. The obvious culprits are the constant common worries about work, money, your family, your health—you know the drill. But there are some more subtle stressors you should be aware of as well.

## It's not the heat, it's the humidity...literally

The climate in which you live can make a substantial difference in the frequency and severity of your attacks. Hot, humid weather in particular is actually a stress factor in and of itself, because (1) heat stresses the body, and (2) air pressure changes from humidity affect the levels of **serotonin** in the body (and over ninety percent of that serotonin is in your

---

[26] Whorwell P.J., et al. "Physiological Effects of Emotion: Assessment via Hypnosis." *Lancet* 340 (11 Jul 1992): 69–72.
[27] Welgan P., et al. "Effect of Anger on Colon Motor and Myoelectric Activity in Irritable Bowel Syndrome." *Gastroenterology* 94, no. 5, pt. 1 (May 1998): 1150–1156.
[28] Levy R.L., et al. "The Relationship between Daily Life Stress and Gastrointestinal Symptoms in Women with Irritable Bowel Syndrome." *J Behav Med* 20, no. 2 (April 1997): 177–193

gut), which in turn reduces your pain tolerance level. You may also find that, personally, some types of weather just stress you out and make you depressed, irritable, or unhappy. It doesn't matter if your preferences seem typical or even logical (maybe you hate blue skies and love drizzle)—what's important is that you consciously note your feelings and physical reactions so that you can deal with them.

While you can't change the weather, of course, you can control where you live. Moving to a different region may sound like a drastic step to take to minimize IBS attacks, but if your local climate is seriously compromising your health you might want to at least consider it. I lived in New England for seven horrendously miserable years and spent every summer battling desperately to maintain stable health in the face of quite literally sickening hot, humid summers. I realized in the end that when I fight my body, my body wins, so I moved back home to the Pacific Northwest where heat and humidity never co-exist. This completely eliminated a serious recurring stress factor from my life. My colon is now much calmer and happier, and so am I. Was the temporary stress of moving worth the permanently beneficial end result? You darn well bet it was.

## Get your Zzzzzsss

The second subtle stress factor that can have a significant impact on IBS symptoms is sleep—or, more accurately, the lack thereof. It's simple common sense that, since a poor night's sleep results in fatigue and a corresponding lower stress-tolerance level, being tired would likely allow IBS to be more easily triggered. But a recent study actually proves this to be so. A significant correlation was noted between morning IBS symptoms and the quality of the previous night's sleep. In fact, morning IBS symptoms seemed to rise or fall in direct association with the prior night's quality of sleep. This is something I've long noticed in my own life. A less strong but still significant relationship was found between end of day IBS symptoms and the quality of sleep during the previous evening.[29] But then, you've probably already discovered this firsthand, haven't you?

---

[29]Goldsmith G., and J.S. Levin. "Effect of Sleep Quality on Symptoms of Irritable Bowel Syndrome." *Dig Dis Sci* 38, no. 10 (1993): 1809–1814.

## FOR CHILDREN WITH IBS

*Stress in childhood is not to be underestimated. Children take their own problems just as seriously as adults take theirs, and they suffer the physical side effects of mental worries as well. For children with IBS, it is crucial that the adults in their lives appreciate and acknowledge the stress they face.*

*This may require special accommodations, particularly since just having IBS can in and of itself be horribly stressful for a child. The disorder is embarrassing enough to many adults, but can be excruciatingly so to kids. They may be extremely uncomfortable telling anyone they have this problem, they might do their best to deny and hide it, and they probably aren't wild about the idea of your telling people either.*

*In fact, parents should not be surprised if their children hide IBS attacks even from them, for several reasons. Just enduring an attack can require privacy and quiet, and discussing the details is likely not the first thing children feel like doing once they've recovered, especially if they already know from experience how suddenly IBS can come and go. They may well want to just put the episode behind them as quickly as possible and move on. Drawing your attention to the attack would prolong the experience—and remember, a child's perception of time is very different from an adult's. To a little kid, ten minutes is a long time and a week can be an eternity. Having to spend just one extra minute dealing with an IBS attack, even in the aftermath, can be truly intolerable from a child's point of view.*

*In addition, if an attack strikes suddenly, your child may simply not have enough time to let you know what's happening (I've had IBS hit me so hard and so fast that I haven't had thirty seconds to make it to the bathroom before the world goes gray and I pass out cold from the pain). If children are in a public place or if there are guests in the home, they may hide the attack from you simply to prevent others from knowing as well. And even though you're their* parent, it might still be horribly embarrassing for them to have to hold a detailed conversation about their bowels with you.

Please respect your child's sensitivities and wish for privacy in this matter. Wait for peaceful times when they're feeling well to discuss the problem with them, and ask specific questions instead of expecting them to volunteer information they may well perceive as humiliating. If they ask you to keep their IBS a secret from certain people or to be vague when discussing the problem, consider humoring them here. There's not much harm in this and the peace of mind it gives your child is well worth the effort on your part.

In practice, this may mean you have to give your child permission to lie, and tell people their illness is something along the lines of food allergies or some generic stomach problem. I would even go so far as to support children who want their parents to lie for them. I know it seems ridiculous to adults, but it may well help your child tremendously to have your reassurance that you will not be discussing their colon in great detail with other people.

I have one particularly vivid memory from the 4th grade, when I first developed IBS, of overhearing my grandmother discussing my symptoms in gory detail with a friend of hers. This happened the day after yet another fruitless and frustrating doctor's appointment about my symptoms, which were completely undiagnosed (my problem had actually been treated so dismissively by my pediatrician that I hold her in contempt to this day).

As soon as my grandmother's friend left, I threw a tantrum out of both fury and humiliation, and the fight ended with my normally unflappable Grams telling me, "Fine! I won't talk about you at all, with any of my friends, ever again!" To which I screamed back, "Fine! I hope that's a promise!" I then ran out of the house, still completely distraught, and didn't come back until I had calmed down. When I came home later, I caught Grams (famous in my family for her honesty and fairness, and for never breaking a promise or revealing a secret) on the phone, talking to yet another friend about my symptoms. It was the one and only time in my life I ever saw an utterly guilty expression on my wonderful grandmother's face.

I can look back now and laugh at this memory, particularly since it's become a family legend as the only time Grams was ever caught red-handed at anything. At the time, however, it was anything but funny. I felt so betrayed and humiliated I refused to speak to my grandmother for the rest of the day. She did apologize and tried her best to explain that she was only trying to help me, but I simply didn't want to hear it. In hindsight, as an adult I realize her intentions were obviously in my best interest. She was as frustrated as I was by my pediatrician's ignorance and incompetence, and she was turning to her friends in hopes of gleaning useful information or finding similar experiences. She was only trying to help any way she could, but it was impossible for me to appreciate this at the time despite the fact that I loved her dearly. The embarrassment of having her friends know about a problem that totally mortified me was just too overwhelming. Was this a rational reaction on my part? No, but I was only nine years old. Sometimes that's a valid excuse.

Just try to keep in mind that your child may also have a similarly strong sense of privacy, and this should be respected whether it makes much sense to you or not. Children are dealing with fears of being teased that adults don't face, and they risk being humiliated by their siblings, friends, or schoolmates in the aftermath of attacks of cramps or diarrhea in a way adults simply won't encounter from other adults. So try to put yourself in their place, and remember your own personal childhood embarrassments (I'll bet some memories are still vivid), and then cater to the sensitivities of your children. If they have IBS they truly need this consideration from you, as they are unlikely to get it from anyone else. Be their ally in the ways they need and ask you to be.

*living*

# Give This a Try— Therapeutic Heat, Meditation, Yoga, and Tai Chi

**FOR DAY-TO-DAY** health maintenance, following the dietary guidelines for IBS will definitely help you weather stressful situations without suffering attacks. However, there are also quite a few options for dealing with stress head-on and thus increasing your ability to manage it successfully.

## Therapeutic heat

*"Heat relaxes everything and makes me feel better immediately."*

—MRS. ANALY ALFONSO, Melbourne, Australia, recently diagnosed IBS Sufferer.

*"I was diagnosed with IBS less than a year ago, though I've been suffering severe abdominal cramps and diarrhea for about four years. I believe the onset of my symptoms is related to my having babies and/or the dysfunction of my thy-*

*roid. When I am premenstrual I am at my worst and most sensitive. Anything will trigger an attack. The use of a heat pack has been the most remarkable discovery I have made. I heat it up in a microwave and place it directly on my lower abdomen, while I lie down and try to relax. What a fantastic help! It has actually stopped my cramps on the spot. The heat relaxes everything and makes me feel better immediately. The hotter the pack the better—if the pack is too hot in some places I just use a small towel underneath. It can go with me wherever I need to be, can be reheated again if it gets cold, and it gives me some security and confidence when going out, which otherwise can be so scary. Alternatively, a hot bath, especially with essential oils in it, can be use- ful too. This is a new discovery for me, but a goody. I'd like to pass it on!"*

Yep, just plain old heat can provide unparalleled relaxation and help prevent stress-related attacks, as well as relieve abdominal cramps once they've already begun. If you have access to a Jacuzzi, steam bath, or sauna, take advantage of this and try engaging in regular sessions of heat-induced bliss. A hot oil massage, especially with aromatherapy, can work wonders too. Make a particular effort to try heat therapy right before any upcoming stressful event— it's a great pre-emptive strike. It doesn't take much effort to try this approach. A simple hot bath will do, or even a long hot shower. You can also wrap yourself up in an electric blanket, or apply a hot water bottle or heat pack directly to your abdomen. Use of a heat pack is particularly beneficial for women when it's used in anticipation of menstrual cramps. Try direct, intense lower abdominal heat the day and night before you expect to be in pain, and odds are you will significantly lessen both your cramps and the likelihood of a related IBS attack.

## *Meditation*

Meditation is a solitary, sedentary practice that deliberately suspends the normal stream of consciousness occupying the mind in order to relax the body and induce mental calm. There are many approaches to meditation, but most involve a concentrated effort to focus on a single peaceful thought, mental image, or sound, with the aim of quieting your mind's "busyness" and achieving a state of tranquility. Meditation should be a sim- ple, natural, and effortless practice during which your external awareness dissipates and you experience a pleasant state of restful alertness, released from stress and fatigue.

Many forms of meditation originated from Eastern religious practices, but simply practicing meditation techniques is a non-religious activity requiring no specific belief system or lifestyle change. Most people find it very easy to learn and it certainly requires no special ability. Meditation is practiced by people of all ages (including children), education levels, cultures, religions, and countries worldwide. It can be appropriate for people of any background.

There are many different approaches to meditation, each with a different name and technique. While they vary in complexity from strictly disciplined practices to general recommendations, all seem to achieve similar physical and psychological benefits. In general, the calming mental exercises of meditation have several elements in common:

- A quiet, peaceful environment for practicing
- A consistent time of day for practice
- A set length of time for practice (often fifteen to twenty minutes, twice daily)
- A comfortable upright, straight-backed position
- A mental focal point of concentration
- Slow, rhythmic breathing
- Eyes closed to turn attention inward
- Physical stillness and passivity

Why should you bother? Well, meditation offers a simple, well-proven means of reducing the risk for or even reversing health problems associated with stress, including: high blood pressure; chronic respiratory problems such as emphysema and asthma; cardiovascular disease; anxiety and panic attacks; mild depression; insomnia; substance abuse; tension migraines; premenstrual syndrome; and, last but not least, IBS.

How is this possible? Meditation has been shown to actually induce physical changes in the body associated with rest and relaxation, including: a rise in the intensity of brain alpha waves characterizing quiet, receptive states; lower levels of stress hormones; improved circulation; lower levels of lactic acid, a by-product of tension and anxiety; reduced oxygen consumption; and a slower heart rate. It's easy to see why health improvements directly follow.

Meditation is also an excellent means for managing chronic pain and achieving pain relief, a top priority for many IBS sufferers. In addition to alleviating the pain itself, meditation also helps people cope with unrelieved pain (and its anticipation) by reducing tension and anxiety. What's interesting is that no one really knows how or why meditation provides pain relief, despite its well-established success rate. Research has suggested several probable mechanisms, however, and their relationship to the type of pain characterized by IBS is striking.

Primarily, the very heart of meditation is relaxation, which indisputably helps relieve and prevent the muscle tension or spasms contributing to (or, in IBS, directly causing) pain. The addition of anxiety, inevitable when people anticipate pain, as IBS sufferers so often do, increases muscle tension further. By relieving that anxiety meditation offers another route to pain relief.[30] In addition, meditation can also alter someone's emotional reaction to pain, a component as important as the physical element. Meditation can simply make pain more bearable, enabling people to successfully live with it and manage it.

This is an important point, because in physiological terms, the physical sensations and emotions associated with pain are processed by different parts of the brain. Meditation may simply allow people to tolerate pain previously perceived as unbearable, by altering the manner in which the brain responds to it. In fact, meditation may actually change the neural pathways that control the physical sensation of pain, by stimulating the inhibitory nerves that extend from the brain to the spinal cord.[31] Given that current IBS research indicates a problem with the processing of gut neural impulses in the brain, and resultant pain, it is easy to see how meditation may well be one of the best strategies for coping with or altogether eliminating IBS attacks.

---

[30] Howard Fields, M.D., University of California, San Francisco. NIH Technology Assessment Panel for Meditation.
[31] Catherine Bushnell, Ph.D, McGill University.

## *Resources*

Most people prefer to take lessons in meditation, and learn it in the context of group practice, but it's possible to teach yourself through books or videotapes. There are no official licensing or certification procedures, or requirements for meditation instructors, and no central directory of practitioners, so if you wish to learn meditation from someone in person you should simply look for a teacher who is experienced, and whose personality and approach you feel comfortable with. Feel free to ask for referrals from other students. To find teachers or classes in your area, check:

Hospitals, clinics, or private medical practices for referrals
Your local yellow pages
Holistic health yellow pages (in many metropolitan areas)
Holistic health centers
Health/metaphysical oriented book stores
Your local gyms
Local continuing education programs

## *For further information contact:*

**Insight Meditation Society**
1230 Pleasant St.
Barre, MA 01005
Phone: 508-355-4378
*www.dharma.org/ims.htm*

**Maharishi Vedic Universities**
Phone: 800-888-5797
*www.maharishi.org*

**Institute of Noetic Sciences**
475 Gate Five Rd., Suite 300
Sausalito, CA 94965
Phone: 415-331-5673
*www.noetic.org*

**Siddha Yoga Meditation Centers**
Phone: 845-434-2000
*www.siddhayoga.org*

**Omega Institute for Holistic Studies**
Phone: 800-944-1001
*www.eomega.org*

**Vipassana Meditation Centers**
Phone: 413-625-2160
*www.dhamma.org*

## Yoga

Yoga is considered a form of moving meditation. It's a term that encompasses over one hundred different disciplines, but yoga (the Sanskrit word for "union") as it is commonly understood refers to *hatha yoga*, a system of physical and mental exercises. Hatha yoga rests on three foundations—exercise, breathing, and meditation—with the goal of joining together the body and mind into a state of balance and harmony. The interplay of these three elements and the studied repetition of each is considered key to achieving their benefits. Most current American hatha yoga practitioners follow a system of eight steps, consisting of:

1. restraint
2. observance
3. physical exercises
4. breathing techniques
5. preparation for meditation
6. concentration
7. meditation
8. absorption

The focus of hatha yoga is typically concentrated on steps 3, 4, and 5. The exercises are a series of prescribed postures. These poses stretch and strengthen muscles, improve posture and the flexibility of the skeletal system, and compress then relax organs and nerves. The intent is to increase the body's physical efficiency and overall health. Typically, each pose will be held for a set period of time, ranging from a few seconds to several minutes. Some postures may be repeated, while others will be performed just once. Many yoga exercises might seem like familiar stretches, while others will be much more complicated. To maintain physical balance and harmony among the muscle groups, the exercises will follow a set order. As you progress through the various postures, you'll move gently and smoothly, without any bouncing or jerking. There will be periods of rest after every few postures. From the simplest to the most difficult poses, the goal remains the same: to easily but thoroughly stretch all of the muscles in the body while gently contracting, releasing, and stimulating the internal organs.

Breathing is slow, deep, and controlled. Yoga breathing techniques are based on the belief that breath is the source of life in the body, and breath control is intended to improve the health and function of both body and mind. Shallow or hurried breathing is considered to have negative physical and mental consequences. During yoga practice you will focus on your breathing, and work through several breathing exercises. You may inhale during certain postures and exhale for others.

You prepare for meditation through the exercises and controlled breathing. Meditation supplements and reinforces the exercise and breathing disciplines, by relaxing the physical body and focusing the mind. The goal is to achieve a quiet, tranquil state of awareness, and the result is reduced stress and increased energy.

Yoga, like meditation, has traditionally been associated with Eastern religious practices. However, any spiritual aspects of yoga are strictly individual, do not require any specific beliefs or faiths, and do not interfere with a person's religious traditions or lack thereof. Yoga is suitable for adults of any age or physical condition, as its approach is non-strenuous in nature. There are even routines offering special techniques for those with health limitations due to illness, injury, obesity, or inactivity. However, yoga as practiced by adults is not always considered appropriate for children under age sixteen, as their bodies are still growing, and the effect of yoga exercises on the glandular and other bodily systems may interfere with their natural development (there are special yoga classes for children, and if you are considering this option I would urge you to find a good local instructor and ask his or her opinion). The more strenuous yoga exercises are not recommended for menstruating women, pregnant women in their first trimester, or nursing mothers.

Yoga has been proven to provide a variety of significant health benefits, both physical and mental. It can help alleviate or manage chronic health conditions, including: back pain, arthritis, depression, diabetes, asthma, migraines, and substance abuse. It has been shown to increase the efficiency of the heart and slow the respiratory rate, lower blood pressure, and contribute to the reversal of heart disease. In terms of overall physical fitness yoga improves posture, muscle fitness, circulation, coordination, range of motion, and flexibility. As a stress management technique yoga is superb; it promotes relaxation, reduces anxiety, improves sleep patterns, and—you knew it was coming—helps stabilize digestion, including IBS symptoms.

> *"I've been practicing yoga for just four months now … and my constipation is gone!"*
>
> —MONIQUE SPENCER, age 25, British Columbia, Canada,
> IBS sufferer since early childhood, undiagnosed until age 19.

*"I've been sick from IBS since I was a young child. When I was thirteen years old, I had to take a year off of school because I was hospitalized for six months of tests in the hopes that someone would figure out what was wrong with me. I never did graduate because I missed so many days and fell too far behind. By the time I was about eighteen, I suffered from diarrhea constantly, and this went on for almost two years. I suffered from dehydration and made numerous trips to the hospital. Then, very quickly, that diarrhea turned to constipation. This was even worse because along with the constipation came* extreme *bloating (to the point where I was rushed to the ER for the pain the pressure caused), nausea (so bad that I feared any movement at all would cause vomiting), gas cramps (excruciatingly sharp pain), and acid reflux. These symptoms lasted for about five years, though I saw just about every specialist, gastroenterologist, and took every test available. In the last eight years I tried over thirty-five different medications that I can remember, in the hopes of controlling the pain and nausea. IBS caused so much stress in my life that for many years I was suicidal. I simply did not want to live like this. Also as a direct result of IBS, I developed a severe case of agoraphobia. Just thinking about leaving the house caused severe panic attacks. I have learned how to control this now, for the most part, but there are still times when, if I'm not feeling well, just going to check the mail is something I have to work up the courage to do.*

*During this time my weight dropped to ninety pounds. Since I could not get to the grocery store, I could not eat. I could not keep a job. Living a life like this prevented me from getting any exercise (all I could do was sleep and cry), and as a result all of my muscles began to hurt. To try and remedy this, and hoping to regain some sanity as well,*

I turned to yoga. I started practicing at home by watching a local television show called Breathingspace Yoga. I followed the program each night at bedtime.

I've been practicing yoga for just four months now, and since I started I have gained back about twenty pounds, which means my weight is once again normal. This is because my appetite has greatly increased. Also, my constipation is gone! When I eat right, my bowel movements are now more regular and normal (which is something they never were before). In the past, eating made my constipation worse, so when I had no money and was too afraid to go to the grocery store, I found to my surprise that this actually helped the pain, because if there was no food for me to digest, there was no constipation. This vicious cycle has ended, though diet can still be a big issue. I do sometimes have to be careful so as to prevent another attack.

When I first started yoga, there was a four or five day period where I had to urinate constantly. As it turned out I was retaining a ton of water from all of my constipation and bloating. This is no longer the case. My skin now looks healthier, too, and I think I have released a lot of toxins from my body. One more thing…I have a disorder with the level of bile produced by my liver. When I am constipated, I can get very jaundiced. Since I started practicing yoga, this is no longer a problem.

I now practice yoga every night before I go to bed, and sometimes in the morning. I also do stretches and certain positions throughout the day as I feel they're needed. For example, if I am having a particularly bad stomach day or cramps, I'll do some positions that are good for the digestive system. I've found that yoga is best done on an empty stomach, and quite often it stimulates my appetite. This is very good, as I am still almost always nauseous.

My typical bedtime routine lasts anywhere from twenty to forty-five minutes, and sometimes an hour. It helps me sleep, and when I have a more restful night, I generally feel better the next day. This is a cycle that I now find essential to my daily life. I feel the effects of my yoga practice immediately if I'm having an attack (it is so relaxing), but it also works as a preventative measure. I do it mostly to relax and because I know that if I do yoga the night before, I'm almost guaranteed to have a better day the next day than if I didn't do any yoga. If I miss a day or two, my IBS attacks seem to be worse, especially the back pain associated with my bowel cramps. If I'm feeling stressed, anxious, *depressed, or if I'm in the middle of a panic attack, any of the inverted yoga positions almost immediately wipe that feeling away. There's something about placing the crown of the skull against the floor that is totally grounding. Letting the blood flow back to the brain is so...I can't even think of the right word...It's pretty amazing. It can just snap me into a good mood and expel my anger and sadness. I am still working at regaining my health overall, but yoga has made a world of difference so far."*

Like meditation, yoga produces measurable physiological changes in the body and an alteration in brain-wave activity reflecting an induced state of deep relaxation, but science cannot yet explain exactly why this is true. Though the beneficial effects of yoga are undisputed, no one quite knows what produces them. Practice may promote the release of endorphins, the body's natural painkillers, or many of the benefits may be the result of physical and mental stress relief. There are currently several studies in progress by the Office of Alternative Medicine at the National Institutes of Health that hope to produce some clear answers on the subject.

For people with IBS, yoga is perhaps most beneficial for its ability to reduce the stress, anxiety, and pain of chronic illness. Regular practice will indisputably improve your physical and mental fitness, promote relaxation, and give you a sense of control over your health and well-being. As with other stress management techniques, the more you practice, the greater your improvement.

## Resources

Yoga is typically taught in group classes, although private instruction may be available. Most people find it easier to learn yoga in person from a qualified instructor, but you can also teach yourself from books or videotapes. Yoga has no special requirements for clothes or equipment, just bare feet. It's recommended that, like meditation, yoga be practiced consistently both in terms of time of day and length of session. An average class is given weekly and lasts about an hour, though shorter sessions can be beneficial if adhered to regularly. You will be expected to practice your routine at home on a daily basis. As with all forms of stress management, consistency and frequency are crucial for obtaining the best results.

There are no standard certification or licensing requirements for yoga instructors. You will need to observe a yoga class before you sign up, looking for a style of teaching and a level of difficulty that appeals to you. Traditionally, the relationship between teacher and student was on a one-to-one basis and taken very seriously by both parties. Advanced yoga practitioners do not take their studies lightly, and at a minimum, a qualified yoga teacher should:

○ Remain an active student and in regular contact with his or her own teacher

○ Practice yoga postures, breathing, and meditation daily

○ Have studied the major yoga texts

○ Practice ethical behavior, conduct classes in a responsible and safe manner, and give each student individual attention.

○ Abstain from smoking, alcohol abuse, and drug use, and follow a healthy diet

○ Have training in basic anatomy and the physical effects of yoga techniques, and the ability to tailor practices according to each student's ability and possible medical restrictions

○ Separate yoga from religion, and never impose his or her own personal beliefs on a student

To find yoga instructors in your area, check:

Your yellow pages
Local gyms and health clubs
YMCA/YWCA
Massage therapists
Alternative healing clinics
Local health food stores
Continuing education classes

A number of reputable yoga schools certify their graduates, and the associations below can supply a list of recognized schools and/or classes in your area.

**American Yoga Association**
Sarasota, FL
Phone: 941-927-4977
*www.americanyogaassociation.org*

**International Association of Yoga Therapists**
Sebastopol, CA
Phone: 707-928-9898
*www.iayt.org*

## Tai Chi

Tai Chi is a traditional Chinese exercise that's considered an internal martial art as well as a healing art and, like yoga, is a type of moving meditation. All Chinese healing arts and martial arts are based upon the theory of the five elements: metal, water, wood, fire, and earth. These elements correspond to many facets in nature, including the five seasons (fall, winter, spring, summer, and Indian summer) and the five main organs of the body (lungs, kidneys, liver, heart, and spleen). The element theory reflects the creation and control of energy (*chi*), in both nature and the body. Metal when heated becomes liquid (water), water nourishes the tree (wood), the tree ignites to make fire, and ashes become earth—this is the five element creation cycle. Metal cuts wood, tree roots hold the earth, earth contains water, water puts out fire, and fire melts metal—this is the five element control cycle.

These metaphors are used in Chinese medicine to help understand imbalances in the body that result in health problems, as the five element processes are seen as paralleling what happens within the body and how organs develop and control energy. Chinese healing arts include Tai Chi, acupuncture (which you'll learn about soon in Day 7), as well as food and herbal medicines (which are often offered in conjunction with acupuncture treatments).[32] All forms of traditional Chinese medicine strive for the same goal—strong, balanced, free-flowing internal energy—using different techniques.

Tai Chi practitioners follow patterns of slow, graceful, precisely controlled movements. Correct posture and breathing control are emphasized, and the fluid motions promote the harmony of body and mind. Tai Chi forms consist of sequential movements of specific positions, one

---

[32] Different foods are believed to correspond to different organs, and can supplement or remove excess energy from these organs. Herbal medicine is treated as food, but herbs are deemed to have stronger qualities. The five elements of foods and herbs are: bitter (heart); sweet (spleen); pungent (lungs); sour (liver); and salty (kidney). For in-depth information about the Chinese five element theory and herbal/food healing, please see Paul Pitchford's *Healing with Whole Foods: Oriental Traditions and Modern Nutrition* (North Atlantic Books, 1993), which also has a terrific bibliography.

flowing smoothly into the other from a set beginning to an end. A single form can include up to one hundred positions and take twenty to thirty minutes to complete, though ten minutes is average. Tai Chi forms can be performed almost anywhere and anytime, by an individual or in a group. Experts recommend practicing at the same time each day, every day, and many teachers will also designate specific times of day as suitable (or not).

Tai Chi is based on the belief that a person's vital energy force, or *chi*, flows through the body along specific meridians, nourishing and sustaining all tissues and organs. Tai Chi experts believe that Tai Chi's health benefits result from a person's balancing the energy of his or her five key organs by eliminating any excesses or deficiencies, and breaking up any blockages in the flow. The origin and center of the body's *chi* is considered to be the *dantien*, an area of the body located right below the navel. All Tai Chi movements originate from the *dantien* and focus on this center of the body's vital force.

Tai Chi necessitates great concentration, erasing everything from your mind so that you can focus on the smooth, gentle movements and feel a mind-body connection. It is a total body exercise involving all the limbs and joints in relaxed continuous movements.

The health benefits of Tai Chi have proven to be substantial.[33] Tai Chi has been shown to increase physical fitness through strength and muscle tone improvements, as well as improve range of motion, flexibility, and coordination. The basic weight-bearing movements help fortify both muscle and bone, and the coordinated movement of body, head, and eyes helps recalibrate the inner ear, improving balance. The low-intensity movements have an aerobic effect on the cardiovascular system, and lower blood pressure, heart rate, and stress levels, while improving circulation. Tai Chi's

---

[33] Tai chi has shown benefits above and beyond traditional exercises, including substantially lower levels of confusion, tension, depression, anger, and fatigue on psychological tests. It may be that Tai Chi's mental discipline—involving visualization, meditation, and focused concentration—reduces stress and provides mental clarity. [See Clinical Psychologist David A. Renjilian's survey of sixty-six athletes at Marywood University in Scranton, PA (thirty-nine participating in martial arts and twenty-seven participating in team sports). *Allure*, March 2001, 130.]

slow, deep breathing induces mental relaxation, increases energy, and improves concentration. The natural extension of the body and limbs improves flexibility and posture. Overall, it is a very low-impact, low-intensity exercise regimen that is appropriate for anyone and particularly beneficial to elderly people.[34]

Tai Chi must be learned from an instructor who has mastered the martial art, and classes are typically taught in weekly sessions. You will learn and memorize the positions of the various forms, and with practice be able to achieve a fluid, well-coordinated, whole-body movement. As you follow the sequence of forms, you will focus on your *dantien*, concentrate on the deep breathing and slow movements of the exercise, and feel a heightened awareness of your body and a clarity of thought and feeling.

There are considered to be five principles of successful Tai Chi practice:[35]

1. Calm down, and think of Tai Chi only.
2. Eliminate any exertion.
3. Be consistent in movement and speed.
4. Practice truly and precisely, studying the movements you make.
5. Persevere. Practice for the same length of time, at the same hour each day.

Although the basic movements of Tai Chi forms can be learned fairly quickly, complete mastery can take a lifetime. The challenge lies in the introspective nature of the exercise: developing your internal energy and feeling the flow as it moves through your body, then detecting and releasing energy blockages to regain the strong, healthy flow of *chi*. This will also allow you to recognize stress and tension in your body, and dissolve them by working through the Tai Chi forms.

As with all types of stress management, the physical and emotional health benefits of Tai Chi are the result of the practice itself, and won't persist once the exercise is stopped. Consider Tai Chi as part of your lifetime lifestyle management of IBS, and try it as a preventative strategy to reduce your risk of attacks by minimizing the impact stress has on your body and life.

---

[34] Tai Chi has been found to significantly reduce the number of falls among elderly practitioners.

[35] Tai Chi grand master Ma Yueh Liang in Bill Moyers's *Healing and the Mind* (Main Street Books, 1995).

## *Resources*

Tai Chi experts emphasize that personalized teaching is necessary to ensure that your movements and posture are correct, so you will need to find a good Tai Chi class in your area. Tai Chi really can't be properly learned from a book or videotape. There is no national certifying organization for Tai Chi instructors, so you will have to make a judgment call when it comes to choosing your own teacher. Visit several different classes, observe the teacher and students, check the instructor's credentials, and ask lots of questions. Check:

Your local yellow pages
Local gyms, community centers, and health clubs
YWCA/YMCA

## *Or contact the following associations:*

**American Association of Acupuncture and Oriental Medicine**
Catasauqua, PA
Phone: 888-500-7999
*www.aaom.org*

**American Foundation of Traditional Chinese Medicine**
505 Beach St.
San Francisco, CA 94133
Phone: 415-776-0502

**East-West Academy of Healing Arts**
San Francisco, CA 94108
Phone: 415-788-2227
*www.eastwestqi.com*

**IN A SENTENCE:**

> *Stress is a powerful trigger for IBS, but lifestyle habits ranging from adequate sleep and a suitable climate to meditation, Tai Chi, and yoga can all work wonders for preventing or minimizing stress-related attacks.*

*task list*

> 1. **TRY TO FIND A DOCTOR YOU CAN ESTABLISH AN ONGOING, HELPFUL RELATIONSHIP WITH REGARDING YOUR IBS.**
>
> 2. **HAVE A TRIAL RUN WITH A PRESCRIPTION MEDICATION FOR YOUR SYMPTOMS, AND REMEMBER THAT IF THE DRUG DOESN'T HELP, THERE ARE MANY OTHER OPTIONS FOR YOU TO TRY.**

# Doctors' Visits and Medical Options

**ALTHOUGH IBS** cannot be managed on a day-to-day basis by a physician (that's up to you), it is important to establish and maintain a good working relationship with the family doctor or gastroenterologist who will be treating your symptoms. This may not be as simple you'd wish.[36] Unfortunately,

---

[36] On average, doctors who treat IBS rate the pain felt by their IBS patients as being significantly less severe than the patients themselves report. Furthermore, a majority of doctors say that while IBS may be distressing, it is not a serious medical condition, despite the fact that three out of ten women with IBS report having been hospitalized for their abdominal symptoms at some point. More than one in four women with IBS say that their doctor does not understand how much pain or discomfort they feel and that there is no point in consulting their doctor about their symptoms. Nearly a third of all U.S. physicians mistakenly believe that IBS is primarily a psychological problem. (Citations from the largest, most comprehensive national survey ever conducted on IBS, July/August 1999, by Schulman, Ronca and Bucuvalas, Inc., funded by GlaxoWellcome.)

the word many IBS patients currently use to describe their relationship with doctors is "frustrating." Although a minority of IBS patients think their physicians are wonderful, most are dissatisfied, and feel that doctors need to better understand IBS and the difficulties it creates in their lives.[37] This is why it is crucial that you feel in partnership with your physician. As you learn how to take responsibility for your health it will be of great assistance to have your doctor's help, support, advice, and understanding in the matter. Your doctor should listen, ask questions, make suggestions, and be empathetic. If your doctor does not view IBS as a legitimate medical disorder and fails to offer enough time to help you take control of your symptoms, you need to find a new doctor.

If you don't have any friends or family members who can recommend a good gastroenterologist, try asking a favorite doctor of yours in a different field whom he or she would consult about IBS. If you've joined a support group (which we'll address in Month 3) see if any of the members are happy with their physicians, or post a request for recommendations from other patients at an internet IBS support board such as *www.helpforibs. com/messageboards/*.

Once you've found a satisfactory doctor and established a good working relationship, he or she should educate you about IBS and treat it as they would any other chronic disorder, with a focus on managing your symptoms. What can you fairly expect your doctor to do?[38]

1. Acknowledge the pain.
2. Hold an empathetic and non-judgmental point of view.
3. Educate and reassure you.
4. Set reasonable goals.
5. Help you, the patient, take responsibility.
6. Know his or her limitations and refer you to specialists if necessary.

I would also add that you can expect a good doctor (especially a gastroenterologist) to be well-informed about the effects of diet and stress on IBS. What you cannot expect from your doctor is a cure. Currently there isn't one.

---

[37] Results from DrugVoice's IBSVoice survey of over two thousand patients, one of the largest and most far-reaching studies of IBS patients ever conducted. [Krauth, Melissa, President, DrugVoice LLC. Update on IBSVoice Panel (23 February 2001).]

[38] Dr. Marvin Schuster, Director of the Marvin M. Schuster Center for Digestive and Motility Disorders at Johns Hopkins Bayview Medical Center, Baltimore, MD.

# Questions to Ask Your Doctor

1.  Do my symptoms truly match those of IBS?
2.  Have you run the diagnostic tests necessary to rule out:

    Colon cancer

    Inflammatory bowel diseases (Crohn's and ulcerative colitis)

    Bowel obstructions

    Diverticulosis

    Gallstones

    Food allergies

    Celiac (a genetic, autoimmune disorder resulting in gluten
      intolerance)

    Bacterial infections

    Intestinal parasites

    Endometriosis

    Ovarian cancer

3.  What prescription drugs do you recommend for me, and why? What if they don't work? What about side effects?
4.  Are there any new medical options for IBS on the horizon?
5.  How should I keep myself informed about current IBS research and breakthroughs?
6.  Should I schedule a follow-up visit with you? When?
7.  What about diet?
8.  What about stress management?
9.  What about alternative therapies?
10. What types of supplements, fiber or otherwise, do you recommend?
11. Do you know of any IBS support groups in my area?
12. Can you recommend any good books or literature on the subject?
13. What do you think is the best way to comprehensively manage my symptoms?

It is really most important to see a doctor for your initial diagnosis. Once it's established that you do in fact have plain old IBS and nothing else, you may well have only a few follow-up visits with your doctor, simply because there is not much medical help available for the disorder. I saw a gastroenterologist once for my initial diagnosis at age sixteen, and it was more than a decade later before I needed a follow-up visit. In the meantime my regular family physicians simply continued my prescription anti-spasmodics without any problems.

However, anytime you have new concerns about your condition, questions about prescription medications, or if you suddenly experience different symptoms, it's time to once again visit a gastroenterologist. We'll be following up further with your doctor in Month 4.

### FOR CHILDREN WITH IBS

*As a parent, you have to walk a fine line when your child visits a doctor for GI tract problems. By necessity you must be intimately involved with your children's health care and deal with their doctors firsthand, but the normal way you'd go about this may be in direct conflict with how your children wish to handle the situation.*

*Children are likely have a very strong preference in one of two ways. They may insist that you stay right next to them throughout the examination and every single diagnostic test that follows, and in this case it's easy to comply. However, your child may instead be much more comfortable talking alone with the doctor and having you out of the room. As well as you think you know your child it's best to not make an assumption here (don't even judge from past doctor's visits—IBS can be a whole different ballgame).*

*It's a good idea to casually ask children if they'd rather you stayed in the waiting room when they see their doctor, and make it clear that you'll understand how they feel (and won't be hurt) if they say yes. It may be difficult to even get a straight answer from your children in this matter. They may be so embarrassed and just plain exhausted by IBS that they'll give whatever answer they think will make you drop the subject as quickly as possible. So approach them at a quiet, low-key time when there's no one else around to overhear, give them a hug, ask them what they'd like your role to be* when they see the doctor, and make it clear that you will let them call the shots here. Anything that can be done to minimize the trauma of the experience will help children tremendously. To them, talking to a doctor at all is likely to be much scarier than it is for an adult. To talk about bowel movements with a doctor is truly a nightmare. Whatever steps you can take to make things emotionally easier will earn you your child's undying gratitude.

I really can't stress enough how embarrassing IBS can be to a child, and having to describe their symptoms in detail to a total stranger while sitting half-naked in a paper gown is very traumatic. For me, having my parents with me in that situation just compounded my humiliation. They were very kind, concerned, and supportive, but their presence took away any last shred of privacy I had left in dealing with the problem. Even as a teenager I was much more comfortable meeting with my doctor and enduring the diagnostic tests alone, though I very much wanted my parents right outside in the waiting room the entire time. Fortunately, they were very understanding in this matter, and helped minimize the stress of the situation for me tremendously. They simply met with the doctor alone when I was through. In this way they stayed well-informed and I felt a little less stripped of all dignity by the whole ordeal.

From the vantage point of an adult, my feelings as a child seem inexplicable and frankly rather strange. Nowadays, I couldn't care less if my parents were with me at the doctor's, and their presence certainly wouldn't seem to be an invasion of privacy but a supportive presence. However, this was definitely not how I felt as a child, and my feelings then, no matter how odd they seem today, were very real. I remember the heat of them quite vividly, and I remain thankful that my parents treated them as legitimate.

Any good doctor will respect children's feelings as well, and make the extra effort necessary to put them at ease. You may want to visit a pediatric gastroenterologist, as a doctor who deals exclusively with children should be more likely to understand their quirks and accommodate them. To this day I am grateful to the doctor who finally diagnosed me at age sixteen, as he requested on his own that my parents wait outside the examining room, and this immediately set me at ease. (In hindsight his actions make me suspect he'd had his share of young patients and knew from experience just how to successfully deal with them). He then told me straight-out that every patient he sees feels embarrassed to be there, and that most people are very reluctant to discuss the type of health problems he deals with every single day. He made it clear that the whole topic was very routine to him, that I had nothing to be embarrassed about, that everything I told him he would take seriously, and he then stressed that he really needed to get detailed information from me or he couldn't help. He asked me very specific, yes-or-no questions to "warm me up" to the topic before expecting me to give full-blown descriptions of my attacks. This was the perfect approach for him to take with me, and your child's doctor should strive to find an approach that works equally well.

*living*

# Trying
# Prescription Drugs

**IF YOU'VE** been following this book from day one of your diagnosis, you've likely now had nearly a week with a new IBS medication that was prescribed for you at that time. Typically, most patients are initially prescribed an anti-spasmodic drug upon diagnosis, though you may have received a low-dose antidepressant or anti-diarrheal instead. There are actually quite a few different prescription medications available for IBS, but their effectiveness can vary greatly from one person to the next.[39]

---

[39] The only critical examination of the efficacy of medical treatments for IBS was conducted in 1988. Measures of efficacy, placebo response, trial length, maintaining blindedness, study designs, and statistical considerations were examined. Of the ninety-three controlled pharmacologic studies reviewed at the time, not a single study offered convincing evidence that any pharmacologic therapy was effective in treating IBS symptoms. Studies looked at a wide range of pharmacologic interventions including antispasmodics, anticholinergic/barbiturate combinations, antidepressants, bulking agents, dopamine antagonists, carminatives, opioids, tranquilizers, phenytoin, timolol, and diltiazem. This does not mean that pharmacologic interventions do not work, only that no intervention has been proven to be effective. [Klein, K.B. "Controlled Treatment Trials in the Irritable Bowel Syndrome: A Critique." *Gastroenterology* 95 (1988): 232–241.]

Which particular drug will work best for you is something you'll most likely have to determine through trial and error. If the first medication you try doesn't help much (or at all), don't be discouraged—there are other options available. Remember that there's no one particular treatment of choice but many different medications to try. You should work in partnership with your doctor to determine which medication best fits your needs. This might take a trial period of a few months and several follow-up visits or phone calls. With any new medication, always make sure you receive the clinical insert about health risks, side effects, and possible drug interactions. You may have to specifically ask the pharmacist for this insert (it will be produced by the drug manufacturer) if you don't receive it with your prescription.

Currently, most IBS patients cite great frustration with the lack of safe, reliable, and effective IBS therapies, and would like to see new options made available to them that would have a greater impact on their problem—especially the ability to prevent symptoms.[40] Unfortunately, for now it's mostly a case of better something than nothing at all. So keep your fingers crossed for new treatments on the horizon.

## For pain

The most frequently prescribed drugs for IBS pain are **anti-spasmodics**. These drugs affect gut motor activity and reduce the colon's response to both eating and stress. Anti-spasmodics are meant to be taken thirty minutes before eating, but they can also be taken whenever needed. Sublingual (dissolve under your tongue) and oral (swallow whole) varieties are available. Typically, anti-spasmodics are prescribed for use four times per day (before each meal and bedtime). Since they have no cumulative effect, however, many patients prefer to take them only as necessary. I have had the best luck with Donnatol. For many years previously I used Pro-Banthine, which is actually a children's drug, though I was not a child at the time and had no idea the drug was not likely to be as effective for adults. Discovering this fact did explain why I was always having

---

[40] Results from DrugVoice's IBSVoice survey of over 2,000 patients, one of the largest and most far-reaching studies of IBS patients ever conducted. [Krauth, Melissa, President, DrugVoice LLC. Update on IBSVoice Panel (23 February 2001).]

to take the maximum dose to see any results. In general, I find soluble fiber supplements, peppermint tea (both of which are dealt with in detail in Month 2), and the IBS diet more beneficial than anti-spasmodics most of the time. As a result I take the drugs quite infrequently, a few pills a month at most. However, if I'm under a great deal of stress I may take them with each meal for a few days straight as I find they work half-decently as a preventative measure, though not at all as a means of stopping an attack once it starts.

Low doses of **antidepressants** can raise the pain threshold for the abdominal cramps of IBS, and they can also either increase or decrease (depending upon the class of drug) the rate of gastrointestinal contractions as well, thus altering bowel function in either direction. Why would antidepressants help IBS? These drugs are meant to affect the uptake of **serotonin**—a **neurotransmitter** directly involved in the development of clinical depression—in the brain. However, the enteric nervous system of the gut is also rich with nerves that contain large amounts of serotonin. In fact, 95% of all serotonin in the body is found in the gut, not the brain. So the effect of antidepressants on the brain is felt as a peripheral result in the gut as well.

It's important to note that the dosage of anti-depressants used for IBS is typically far lower than that of the drug when used for depression. It is also crucial that the doctor prescribing this type of drug be very familiar with its use for IBS, as different classes of anti-depressants have varying side effects, and some can greatly worsen, instead of help, IBS symptoms, depending on the patient.

In particular, SSRI anti-depressants (Prozac, Celexa, Zoloft, and Paxil) stimulate serotonin production and can trigger severe IBS attacks in diarrhea-predominant patients, but they may be helpful for constipation. Conversely, tricyclic anti-depressants (such as Elavil) have the best track record of success for reducing diarrhea-predominant IBS symptoms, but patients with constipation are usually not treated with these drugs because of the possibility of exacerbating this symptom. Tricyclic anti-depressants tend to be anticholinergic—that is, they block the activity of the nerves responsible for gut motion. The long-term consequences of taking low-dose anti-depressants for IBS are unknown, and this is a matter that should be discussed with your physician.

**Narcotic analgesics** are opioid drugs and can be highly effective painkillers. One of their chief side effects, constipation, is actually of benefit to some IBS sufferers. Narcotics also induce a feeling of tranquility and promote drowsiness, both of which can be helpful for relieving stress-related attacks. The chief problem with narcotic drugs is that it's next to impossible to get a doctor to prescribe them for you. Although there is mounting evidence that these painkillers are not nearly as habit-forming as previously thought, from your doctor's point of view the risks of addiction are still likely to take precedence over your pain. You'll have to decide for yourself, based on the severity of your symptoms, what your own priorities are in the matter and, if appropriate, try to find an understanding physician. Narcotic painkillers work best on an empty stomach and may take up to an hour to halt an attack. They should only be used in the advent of severe pain that occurs despite dietary and stress management precautions, and should not be used as a preventative measure or on a regular ongoing basis as they can be addictive. In addition, the less frequently this medication is used the more effective it tends to be. On a personal note, when I am struck by a severe attack out of the blue, something that happens several times a year, a prescription narcotic painkiller (typically Vicodin) is the only avenue of help that works for me. I don't have as much luck as I'd like with the drug quickly stopping an attack outright (though I would give anything for this), but it does work beautifully to prevent recurring attacks and allow me to stabilize. It somehow seems to push a "reset button" for my body that breaks the cycle of pain, lets me rest and recover, and from that point on take charge of my health once again through diet and stress management. I only use a handful of these painkillers each year, but when I do need them it's hard to convey the sheer gratitude I feel for their availability.

## For diarrhea

Imodium and Lomotil are the most common anti-diarrheal medications for IBS. They enhance intestinal water absorption, strengthen anal sphincter tone, and decrease intestinal transit, thereby increasing stool consistency and reducing frequency. Both are meant to be used for prevention of diarrhea by taking them prior to events (meals or stress) which typically trigger symptoms. They should be taken with plenty of fresh water. Imodium can be used as a daily maintenance drug, but Lomotil is chemically related to narcotics, and as such is not an innocuous drug, so dosage recommendations should be strictly adhered to (especially in children). Lomotil can be habit-forming, and an overdose could be fatal.

## For constipation

There are no common prescription drugs for constipation-predominant IBS. The use of chemical laxatives (such as Milk of Magnesia or ExLax), which tend to stimulate the bowel by causing an irritated lining, is not recommended as they can easily lead to dependency and they're harmful to the colon. The most typical treatment for constipation is a non-prescription soluble fiber supplement such as Metamucil, Citrucel, or Fibercon (discussed in depth in Month 2), lots of fresh water, and exercise. Unfortunately, this is simply not enough for many people with IBS, but there are currently several research studies underway for a prescription medication that can address the problem safely and effectively.

## Lotronex

Lotronex is a special case when it comes to IBS prescription drugs. Manufactured by GlaxoSmithKline, the FDA approved Lotronex in February 2000 after giving it an expedited, "fast track" review.[41] It was the first of a new generation of agents being studied specifically for the treatment of multiple symptoms of IBS, and it was meant to be prescribed only for women who were diarrhea-predominant.

In clinical terms, Lotronex was a potent and selective 5-HT3 antagonist. In brief, the neurotransmitter serotonin and 5-HT3 receptors that are extensively distributed on enteric neurons in the human GI tract are thought to play a role in increasing the sensation of pain and affecting bowel function in patients with IBS. While the precise mechanism of action of Lotronex was never fully understood, one hypothesis was that

---

[41] The U.S. Food and Drug Administration has reported that average approval time for all new prescription drugs has shrunk from thirty months eight years ago to twelve months today, with high-demand medicines racing to market in as little as six months. Years ago, when Europe took the lead in marketing new drugs, American regulators watched for side effects before approving drugs here. Now, the majority of new drugs worldwide debut in the United States. With this change comes serious risks, as ten drugs have been recalled in America for toxic effects since 1997.

Lotronex blocks the action of serotonin at 5-HT3 receptor sites in the enteric nervous system, thus slowing colonic transit time and preventing IBS diarrhea-predominant symptoms.

In plain English, Lotronex somehow affected the action of serotonin (a neurotransmitter found in abundance in the gut), thus preventing painful cramps and slowing colon contractions to reduce diarrhea. For some patients, Lotronex was quite literally a wonder-drug.

> *"After two weeks of taking Lotronex,*
> *I had my life back!"*

—MELISSA D. GODWIN, Parkersburg, West Virginia,
age 27, IBS Sufferer for 8 years.

*"I have suffered from Irritable Bowel Syndrome for eight years now, and they have been the most miserable years of my life. The symptoms of IBS that I suffer from are: diarrhea, bowel cramping, severe gas, headaches, fatigue, muscle weakness, and sharp stabbing pains in my lower abdomen. Nearly every day, I feel physically and emotionally drained. IBS is not life threatening, but it is life prohibiting. It is difficult to go out to dinner with friends or family because all through dinner, I worry that what I just ate is going to make my bowels cramp. Or, if I go to a movie after dinner I have to sit in the aisle seat in case I have to run off to the rest room. Traveling is nearly impossible. What if I am in the car, nowhere near a rest area, and have that dreaded urgency and cramping? I generally have panic attacks by the time I get out of town. I not only have to be concerned with traveling and public places—this condition affects my job as well. I have tried diet modification, fiber, numerous over-the-counter medications, stress control, anti-depressants, anti-anxiety drugs, and anti-spasmodic medications just to stop the IBS pain. Of all these medications, only one worked. Everything was solved by one little blue pill called Lotronex. After two weeks of taking Lotronex, I felt like a new person. I had my life back! I was able to go to public places and travel. I could eat and drink anything I wanted and I had no cramps, no urgency, and no gas pain. Those were the happiest months of my life! Then Lotronex was pulled off the market, and this was a tragedy to me. The loss of Lotronex led me to the Lotronex Action Group, and I decided to join their fight. I*

*was so thankful they gave me the opportunity to tell my story, because
without Lotronex, I feel like I'm right back where I was before."*

For other patients, however, Lotronex was not a dream but a nightmare. While clinical trials of the drug showed few side effects, reports of serious and even deadly adverse reactions to the medication began cropping up shortly after its FDA approval. In some patients the drug caused side effects so severe they resulted in hospitalization and even death. Through the end of the year 2000, sixty-three patients taking Lotronex developed ischemic colitis, an interruption of the blood supply to the large intestine which results in severe internal damage. Seventy-five patients experienced severe constipation. Most of the patients who developed these problems required hospitalization. In all, the FDA has on record 141 cases of severe gastrointestinal complications in patients who took the drug, and five deaths.[42] As a result of these problems, Lotronex was pulled from the U.S. market in November 2000, just nine months after it debuted.

In response, a group of IBS patients who had experienced great success with Lotronex formed the Lotronex Action Group, a non-profit patient group seeking renewed access to the drug.[43] The Lotronex Action Group believes Lotronex to be safe if dispensed properly, and that the benefits of Lotronex far outweigh the potential risk for adverse side effects. The LAG has urged the FDA not to lose sight of the patients, and to realize that the medical community has been slow to recognize IBS as a legitimate disorder that can have debilitating side affects. The LAG wants taken into account their concerns that efforts for reintroduction of the only effective treatment for some IBS patients suffering from severe diarrhea and abdominal pain will be derailed due to a lack of understanding of the severity of the symptoms IBS can cause. The LAG also

---

[42] Public Citizen, Health Research Group. 1600 20th St. NW, Washington, DC 20009, 202-588-1000, *www.publiccitizen.org.*
[43] Lotronex Action Group, *www.lotronexactiongroup.org.* Tom Bell, Coordinator. Richard Fireman, Coordinator. Corey Miller, Coordinator. Jeffrey Roberts, www.helpforibs.com/messageboards/. The Lotronex Action Group was organized by members of the IBS Self Help Group and former Lotronex users. The Lotronex Action Group is not affiliated with, nor does it receive any funding from, any pharmaceutical company.

maintains that although claims have been made that severe side effects have been linked to Lotronex, it appears that less than a fraction of one percent of the three hundred thousand people taking the drug were affected. Moreover, the LAG contends that no data has been released proving that those who suffered from side effects were ever properly diagnosed with IBS and were also good candidates for Lotronex in the first place.

The Lotronex Action Group has lobbied the FDA for immediate re-release of Lotronex while avenues for continued marketing are explored between the manufacturer, GlaxoSmithKline, and the Food and Drug Administration. Moreover, the LAG ultimately seeks permanent access and safe distribution of the medicine to those diagnosed with diarrhea-predominant IBS.

In response to the pressure from both the pharmaceutical industry and the Lotronex Action Group, the FDA is, as of mid-2001, considering putting Lotronex back on the market. However, any re-introduction may be limited to patients who have previously used it and have not experienced adverse effects, and who have been given an informed consent sheet explaining the potential dangers of the drug. In addition, a registry of all patients taking the drug and their physicians would be kept so the patients can be closely monitored. In the view of Public Citizen, "If anything other than this approach is used, the toll of needless deaths and serious injuries and the repeat ban that will inevitably occur will be on the hands of those FDA officials responsible for such a reckless remarketing."[44]

If nothing else, the Lotronex debacle points out the gaping chasm that remains between the medical needs of IBS patients and the limited drug choices currently available to them.

---

[44] Public Citizen, Health Research Group. 1600 20th St. NW, Washington, DC 20009, 202-588-1000, *www.publiccitizen.org*.

## Medications for IBS

| Medication Class | Examples | Principal Indication | Side Effects and Comments |
|---|---|---|---|
| Antispasmodics | Donnatol (belladonna/phenobarbital) Bentyl (Dicyclomine hydrochloride), Levsin/Levbid (Hyoscyamine sulfate) | Pain and diarrhea | Dry mouth and eyes, urinary retention, tachycardia, drowsiness. Can be mildly constipating. |
| Antidiarrheals | Imodium, Kaopectate, and Maalox (all Loperamide); Lomotil (diphenoxylate and atropine sulfate), Pepto Bismol (bismuth subsalicylate) | Diarrhea, urgency, incontinence | Considerable variation in required dose; can induce constipation, drowsiness and/or dizziness. |
| Tranquilizer/antispasmodic | Librax (Chlordiazepoxide hydrochloride, Clidinium bromide) | Pain, diarrhea | Blurred vision, drowsiness, can be habit-forming. |
| Tricyclic antidepressants | Secondary amines (e.g., nortriptyline, desipramine) Tertiary amines (e.g., amitriptyline, imipramine) | Pain, diarrhea, other discomforts | Fewer CNS and anticholinergic side effects and less sedation, orthostatic hypotension and weight gain with secondary amines; start low and work up to target dosage. Constipation can worsen. |

| Medication Class | Examples | Principal Indication | Side Effects and Comments |
|---|---|---|---|
| Narcotic analgesics | Vicodin (Hydrocodone), Percodan and Percocet (Oxycodone), Demerol (Meperidine), Codeine, Morphine. | Pain, diarrhea | Drowsiness, dizziness, constipation, nausea. Can be habit-forming. Possible dangerous interactions with other prescription and over-the-counter drugs, and alcohol. |
| Newer antidepressants | SSRIs (e.g., fluoxetine, paroxetine) Others (e.g., buproprion, venlafaxine) | Can be used for pain management and constipation in patients who are intolerant to TCAs | Transient exacerbation of nausea; diarrhea can occur with SSRIs; sleep disruption occurs with some agents. |
| 5-HT3 antagonist | Alosetron (LOTRONEX) | Affects multiple symptoms in diarrhea-predominant female patients only, including pain, urgency, and diarrhea. | Effectiveness has not been shown in men. Lotronex was withdrawn from the market in the U.S. in November 2000. |
| Under investigation | Cilansetron | 5-HT3 antagonist | Under investigation by Solvay Pharmaceutical for chronic diarrhea. |
| | Prucalopride | 5-HT4 receptor | Under investigation by Janssen Research Foundation for chronic constipation. |
| | Zelnorm (tegaserod) | Constipation | In development by Novartis for abdominal pain or discomfort and constipation in women. FDA approval anticipated 2002/2003. |

**IN A SENTENCE:**

> *It's crucial to see a competent, sympathetic doctor to ensure you've been properly diagnosed with IBS and have a resource for answers to all of your medical questions, but after your diagnosis the daily management of symptoms will probably stem more from lifestyle changes than any currently available prescription drug.*

*learning*

*task list*

1. CHOOSE AN ALTERNATIVE THERAPY AND
   MAKE AN APPOINTMENT FOR YOUR FIRST
   TREATMENT.

# Alternative Therapies and How They Can Help

GIVEN THAT IBS is a dysfunction, not a disease, and a severely under-researched one at that,[45] it's easy to see why there is a shortage of highly effective and safe medical options for treatment. Just as the disorder must be managed through lifestyle modifications such as diet and stress reduction, both non-traditional approaches to treating illness, so there is another avenue of addressing IBS that is currently outside, but gaining widespread acceptance in, medical practice. This is the use of alternative therapies, particularly acupuncture

---

[45] IBS receives less than one percent of digestive disease research funding through the National Institutes for Health, despite the fact that it is the single most common digestive disorder diagnosis in America (International Foundation for Functional Gastrointestinal Disorders).

and hypnotherapy. Both forms of treatment can (and should) be tailored to specifically address IBS patients, with a focus on reducing the frequency, severity, and duration of attacks. Impressively high success rates are achievable, and side effects should be non-existent. Interested?

*living*

# Acupuncture and Hypnotherapy

## Acupuncture

ACUPUNCTURE, LIKE Tai Chi, is one of the ancient forms of traditional Chinese healing arts. Unlike Tai Chi, however, acupuncture is not a self-directed therapy, whereby a person balances his or her own body's *chi* (energy or life force). Acupuncture is instead a treatment administered to a patient by a trained practitioner, who balances the body's *chi* by stimulating areas (acupuncture points) along the primary meridians, or channels, through which *chi* flows. These meridians run deep within the body and regulate all physical and mental processes, surfacing at the various acupoints. Acupuncture is the stimulation or sedation of these acupoints in order to balance the body's flow of *chi*.

The traditional Chinese perspective on acupuncture reflects the belief that the body is a complex and holistic physical/mental/emotional/spiritual system, balanced between health and sickness in a constantly changing flow of energy. According to this viewpoint, imbalances in this natural energy flow are thought to cause disease. Acupuncture, frequently in conjunction with the use of Chinese herbal and/or food medicine, restores health by balancing and improving the flow of *chi*, restoring proper function of muscles, nerves, vessels, glands, and organs.

An acupuncture treatment will strengthen the flow of *chi* or remove blockages in the meridians via the insertion of very thin, flexible acupuncture needles, from a depth of just beneath the skin to about an inch, at various acupoints along the meridians. (Please note that it's important to ask and verify that your acupuncturist works solely with single-use, sterile, disposable needles, as one of the only real (though rare) risks of acupuncture is infection or transmission of contagious diseases, such as Hepatitis B, at the puncture site.)

Thousands of these points exist in the body, and each one is associated with a specific internal organ or organ system. As the acupuncture needles are inserted into the acupoints the patient may feel nothing, or a sensation of tingling, aching, warmth, or heaviness. Most people report no pain from the needles, just an odd or unusual physical sensation that is different but not unpleasant. From one to twenty needles may be used in a single treatment session, and often the needles are stimulated after insertion by being twisted or heated with a moxibustion stick of smoldering herbs. This will heighten the sensation of *chi*. Most individual sessions lasts anywhere from about five to sixty minutes, depending on the condition being treated as well as the patient's response to the acupuncture. Typically the needles remain in place for twenty to forty minutes.

The number and frequency of treatments will vary with both the practitioner and the illness being addressed, but may range from a single session to several appointments a week, possibly over a period of several months. In general, for pain relief, six sessions should result in measurable results,[46] and if relief is not obtained after ten sessions the treatment should be deemed ineffective. A credible acupuncturist will recognize treatment failure and will not recommend a continuation of therapy. Treatments often become less frequent over time as the condition subsides, though maintenance sessions may be indicated at various intervals. If your condition is chronic and has been for a long period of time (not exactly unheard of for IBS), you may require regularly scheduled treatments over several months.

[46]NIH Panel.

Both the National Institutes of Health Consensus Panel[47] and the World Health Organization,[48] using different criteria, have identified many different conditions as appropriate for acupuncture treatments, including several that directly pertain to IBS:

O abdominal pain
O muscle cramping
O constipation
O diarrhea

In addition, acupuncture has also been deemed effective as a means of stress reducing and addressing related problems that are often triggers for IBS symptoms, such as:

O anxiety
O insomnia
O nervousness
O menstrual cramps
O premenstrual syndrome

At least one study has directly investigated the use of acupuncture versus relaxation therapy in IBS patients.[49] This research found that patients' quality-of-life and gastrointestinal symptom scores were equally improved in both groups, with a statistically significant reduction in abdominal pain. However, when the patients were followed for a four-week period post-trial period, only in the acupuncture group did pain reduction persist. Furthermore, a significant reduction in stress perception was also observed in the acupuncture group, but not in the relaxation group. The conclusion drawn was that acupuncture is an effective form of treatment for IBS, particularly the pain and stress symptoms, and that its benefits exceed those of standard relaxation treatment.

---

[47] Acupuncture. National Institutes of Health. Consensus Statement 1997 Nov 3–5; 15(5):1–34.
[48] World Health Organization. Viewpoint on acupuncture. Geneva, Switzerland: World Health Organization, 1979.
[49] In a randomized, controlled trial of twenty-seven patients with IBS diagnosed by their own criteria, the study treated the patients with acupuncture or relaxation sessions three times a week for a period of two weeks. A follow-up observation run was then performed for four weeks. (Lu, B., Y. Hu, and S. Tenner. "A Randomized Controlled Trial of Acupuncture for Irritable Bowel Syndrome." Abstract in *Program and Abstracts of the 65th Annual Scientific Meeting of the American College of Gastroenterology* [2000].)

While it is unquestionable that acupuncture can provide significant pain relief and help minimize other symptoms of IBS as well, from a Western medical standpoint (though certainly not from the traditional Chinese medicine point of view) no one quite knows how or why this is true. From the Western viewpoint, it may be that acupuncture affects the nervous system by stimulating the release of endorphins, naturally produced chemicals in the body that block pain signals in the brain and spinal cord. Research has shown that acupuncture results in changes in the conduction of electromagnetic signals in the brain, an alteration of blood circulation within the brain that increases blood flow to the thalamus (the area associated with relaying pain and other sensory impulses), and measurable differences in the brain's output of neurotransmitters such as serotonin, norepinephrine, and of inflammation-causing substances such as prostaglandins.

Why these changes occur is still considered a mystery by doctors and scientists who do not hold with the Chinese concept of *chi*. However, if you're suffering from chronic pain and associated diarrhea or constipation as a result of IBS, odds are you don't care why acupuncture works—just that it *does* work. It's the end result that counts here, not the underlying reasons for success.

On a related note, you've probably noticed by now that many of the most effective treatments for IBS, from meditation to Tai Chi to acupuncture, have well-established and measurable success rates, but no explanation behind their impressive results. You may be intrigued, you may not care. Personally, I am more than willing to give the benefit of the doubt to the concept of *chi* and simply accept that, for whatever reasons, these practices are truly effective. I have also been quite unimpressed by the Western approach to IBS, which until very recently dismissed it outright as a psychosomatic problem, and has not yet even come close to thoroughly understanding the underlying dysfunction or developing an effective form of treatment for it—let alone finding a cure. What matters most to me, and probably to you too, is results. So if something helps prevent or alleviate an IBS attack, then it is by definition a valid form of health care for this disorder. While it's certainly preferable to be able to ask and understand the reasons behind a treatment's effectiveness, in these circumstances it fortunately isn't required in order to reap the benefits (though I remain curious).

Still trying to decide if acupuncture is for you? Precautions are only necessary with this treatment if:

○ You have an uncontrolled bleeding disorder, or are taking an anti-coagulant medication such as Coumadin (warfarin). Acupuncture needles do have the potential to draw blood.

○ You are pregnant. The stimulation of certain acupuncture points, particularly those on or near the abdomen, can trigger uterine contractions and could induce premature labor and possibly miscarriage. Tell your acupuncturist if you are pregnant or even just think you may be.

○ You have diabetes. Acupuncture should be used on your limbs only with extreme caution, as even small skin punctures in a person with diabetic neuropathy can result in severe infections. If you have any concerns in this area consult your physician.

○ You have breast or other implants. Do not have needles placed in the area of the implant.

## Resources

There are currently an estimated thirteen thousand licensed and certified acupuncturists in the U.S. Thirty-five states and the District of Columbia require non-physician acupuncturists to be licensed, but standards vary widely—from minimal to stringent. In unregulated states acupuncture is technically illegal unless performed by a medical doctor, but physicians are permitted to practice acupuncture with little to no training at all.

There is also a confusing array of acupuncture licenses and degrees, including:

○ Doctor of Acupuncture (DAc)
○ Doctor of Oriental Medicine (DOM or OMD)
○ Master of Science in Oriental Medicine (MSOM)
○ Master in Oriental Medicine (MTCM)
○ Master of Science in Oriental Medicine (MSTCM)
○ Licensed Acupuncturist (LAc or LicAc)
○ Registered Acupuncturist (RAc)
○ Certified Acupuncturist (CA)

Because licensing requirements vary so, it can be difficult to judge the credentials of an acupuncturist. This is why it is very important to get a referral for an acupuncturist in your area from a reputable acupuncture organization, such as those listed below.

Take into account the fact that even a licensed, well-credentialed, and experienced acupuncturist might not be particularly talented. If you are unimpressed with the results from your treatments, you may want to at least consider trying a second round of therapy with a new practitioner. You've probably seen several different medical doctors for your IBS, with widely varying degrees of satisfaction from the outcomes of your visits. If acupuncture interests you it's a good idea to put the same time and effort into finding a worthwhile practitioner. The risk is certainly negligible and the rewards may well be great.

## Acupuncture organizations

There are several major national organizations that represent the diversity of thought and traditions within the acupuncture profession in the U.S. Each of these is independent from the others, has a separate mission and role, and works in its own way to support the acceptance of acupuncture based on sound standards of competency. They are:

**National Commission for the Certification of Acupuncturists and Oriental Medicine (NCCAOM)**
Phone: 202-232-1404 or 703-548-9004
*www.nccaom.org*
This group provides certification for practitioners of acupuncture.

The NCCAOM promotes nationally recognized standards of competence for acupuncture and Oriental medicine. NCCAOM certification is used as the basis for licensing in ninety percent of the states that have set standards of practice for acupuncture. Certification in acupuncture is based on a candidate's ability to meet eligibility standards of education and/or experience; passage of the comprehensive written and practical examination; successful completion of an NCCAOM approved Clean Needle Technique Course; and commitment to the professional code of ethics.

All diplomates undergo a recertification process every two years based on criteria that reflect competency to practice a health care profession and that demonstrate continued activity and current knowledge in the field.

The NCCAOM is a member of the National Organization of Competency Assurance and certified by the National Commission for Certifying Agencies, the agency with the highest voluntary standards of certifying agencies in the U.S.

### Accreditation Commission for Acupuncture and Oriental Medicine (ACAOM)
Phone: 301-608-9680
This group sets standards for acupuncture schools and can provide a list of accredited institutions.

The Commission acts as an independent body to evaluate first professional master's degree and first professional master's level certificate and diploma programs in acupuncture and first professional master's degree and first professional master's level certificate and diploma programs in Oriental medicine with concentrations in both acupuncture and herbal therapy for a level of performance, integrity, and quality that entitles them to the confidence of the educational community and the public they serve.

The Commission establishes accreditation criteria, arranges site visits, evaluates those programs that desire accredited status and publicly designates those programs that meet the criteria.

The Commission is recognized by the U.S. Department of Education and the Commission on Recognition of Postsecondary Accreditation and is a charter member of the Association of Specialized and Professional Accreditors.

### Acupuncture and Oriental Medicine Alliance (Acupuncture Alliance)
Phone: 253-851-6896
The Acupuncture Alliance is the national professional membership association founded to represent the diversity of acupuncture practitioners in the US.

The Alliance is committed to:

○ fostering high quality health care, education and research;
○ integrating acupuncture and Oriental medicine into the American health care system;

○ expanding public understanding of the profession; and

○ promoting and cultivating discussion, broad representation and empowerment of members at organizational, state, regional and national levels.

**American Academy of Medical Acupuncture (AAMA)**
Phone: 800-521-2262
This is a telephone referral service for acupuncturists who are also medical doctors.

**American Association of Acupuncture and Oriental Medicine (AAAOM)**
Phone: 610-266-1433
This group can provide nationwide referrals for licensed or registered practitioners.

**National Acupuncture and Oriental Medicine Alliance (NAOMA)**
Phone: 253-851-6896
*www.acuall.org*
This group provides general information on acupuncture and referrals by mail for state licensed or nationally certified acupuncturists.

## *Hypnotherapy*

Hypnotherapy has been approved by the American Medical Association as a valid medical treatment since 1958, though the concept of using a state of hypnosis to alleviate both physical and mental ills has recurred throughout the history of medicine from ancient times. By reaching the subconscious level of the mind, hypnotherapy can be used to alter the way a person consciously perceives health problems and promote new manners of response to them. Hypnosis is often thought to be therapy that only affects the mind, but as mind and body are inseparably joined, hypnosis can also help physical ailments. During a state of hypnosis, consciousness is not lost. It becomes more selective, and typically a patient becomes aware of internal processes rather than the outside world's distractions. Most people report the actual experience of being hypnotized as pleasant, comfortable, and extremely relaxing.

Hypnotherapy is beneficial not only for the relaxation it induces, but for the state of suggestibility that characterizes it. In this state, the mind is open to receiving ideas and suggestions that promote positive thoughts and healing changes.[50] During normal waking hours, the window between

---

[50] It's important to note that only positive suggestions produce results, as it is well-established that a person in a state of hypnosis cannot be made to do anything against his or her will, conscience, or moral values. Even while hypnotized the patient (not the therapist) remains in full control.

the conscious and subconscious minds is closed, but any state of relaxation that results in alpha brain waves will open it. Typically, this happens during sleep, and dreams result. Hypnotherapy induces this same state of relaxation while the patient is awake, and allows helpful suggestions (such as those aimed at controlling health problems) to be directed into the subconscious mind.

Only ten percent or so of the population is not susceptible to hypnosis—the rest of us can turn to this therapy for relief of symptoms from disorders as wide-ranging as: asthma, allergies, strokes, multiple sclerosis, Parkinson's disease, cerebral palsy, high blood pressure, nausea and vomiting, irregular heartbeat, muscle spasms, paralysis, and, with well-documented success rates, Irritable Bowel Syndrome.

Hypnotherapy has in fact proven highly effective in alleviating all of the various IBS symptoms.[51] Over fifteen years of solid scientific research has demonstrated hypnotherapy as an effective, safe, and inexpensive choice for IBS symptom alleviation.[52] It has been so overwhelmingly successful in this regard that Adriane Fugh-Berman, M.D., chair of the National Women's Health Network in Washington, D.C., has said that hypnosis should be the treatment of choice for IBS cases which have

---

[51] In one recent study, Dr. Olafur S. Palsson and colleagues at the Eastern Virginia Medical School in Norfolk, Virginia, provided twenty-four IBS patients, fifteen women and nine men, with seven sessions of hypnosis treatment. In addition, the patients used hypnosis audiotapes at home. At the end of the fourteen-week study period, twenty-one of the twenty-four patients "rated themselves improved in all central IBS symptoms after treatment," the researchers report. Significant improvement was found in abdominal pain, bloating, stool consistency, and bowel movement frequency. Palsson's group also measured the autonomic nervous system, which regulates the digestive system and other involuntary body activities. After the course of hypnotherapy, the autonomic nervous system was less easily stimulated. The researchers propose that this calming effect "may plausibly contribute to the symptom improvement." [Palsson, O., M. Turner, and D. Johnson. "Hypnotherapy for Irritable Bowel Syndrome: Symptom Improvement and Autonomic Nervous System Effects." Abstract in *Program and Abstracts of Digestive Disease Week 2000* 997 (2000).]

[52] One of the earliest studies of hypnotherapy in IBS patients tracked fifty patients, all of whom had been diagnosed with severe intractable Irritable Bowel Syndrome, for a mean duration of eighteen months. Of these patients, divided into three categories of classical cases, atypical cases, and cases exhibiting significant psychopathology, the response rates were 95%, 43%, and 60% respectively. Patients over the age of fifty years responded very poorly (25%) whereas those below the age of fifty with classical Irritable Bowel Syndrome exhibited a 100% response rate. This study confirmed the successful effect of hypnotherapy. [Whorwell, P.J., A. Prior, and S.M. Colgan. "Hypnotherapy in Severe Irritable Bowel Syndrome: Further Experience. *Gut* 28, no. 4 (April 1987): 423–425.]

not responded to conventional therapy. Since the "conventional therapy" offered to most IBS patients ranges from nothing at all to a lifetime prescription for semi-effective anti-spasmodic drugs, I take this statement as the closest thing to a whole-hearted endorsement an alternative therapy can hope to get from a mainstream medical spokesperson.

For IBS, one of hypnotherapy's greatest benefits is its well-established ability to reduce the effects of stress. Your state of mind can have a direct impact on your physical well-being, even when you're in the best of health. If you're struggling with IBS, the tension, anxiety, and depression that comes from living with an incurable illness can actually undermine your immune system and further compromise your health. Hypnotherapy can reduce this stress and its resultant negative impact by placing you in a deeply relaxed state, promoting positive thoughts and coping strategies, and clearing your mind of negative attitudes.

IBS in fact is almost uniquely suited to treatment by hypnotherapy, for several reasons. First, as just noted, stress-related attacks can be significantly reduced. Second, one of the most impressive aspects of hypnotherapy, and of tremendous benefit to IBS sufferers, is its well-documented ability to relieve virtually all types and degrees of pain.[53] Finally, because IBS is not a disease at all but a syndrome, if you can relieve and prevent the symptoms, you have effectively cured yourself of the disorder. The underlying dysfunction may still be present but if you suffer no noticeable effects from it, you will be living an IBS-free life. This outcome is a definite possibility from hypnotherapy treatments.

---

[53] Despite the fact that the neural mechanisms underlying the modulation of pain perception by hypnosis remain obscure, its effects are definitely real. One recent study, using positron emission tomography to identify the brain areas in which hypnosis modulates cerebral responses to a noxious stimulus found that noxious stimulation caused an increase in regional cerebral blood flow in the thalamic nuclei and anterior cingulate and insular cortices. The hypnotic state induced a significant activation of a right-sided extrastriate area and the anterior cingulate cortex. The interaction analysis showed that the activity in the anterior (mid-)cingulate cortex was related to pain perception and unpleasantness differently in the hypnotic state than in control situations. The result? Hypnosis decreased both pain sensation and the unpleasantness of noxious stimuli. Conclusions? Both intensity and unpleasantness of the noxious stimuli are reduced during the hypnotic state. In addition, hypnotic modulation of pain is mediated by the anterior cingulate cortex. [Faymonville, M.E., et al. "Neural Mechanisms of Antinociceptive Effects of Hypnosis." *Anesthesiology* 92, no. 5 (May 2000):1257–1267.]

As with other alternative therapies, though there is solid evidence that hypnotherapy can provide lasting health benefits for many patients, there is uncertainty about precisely how and why the treatments work. Most scientists believe that hypnotherapy acts upon the unconscious, and affects the body's regulation of involuntary reactions that are normally beyond a person's control. Hypnotherapy puts these autonomic responses under the patient's power. Happily, treatment is suitable for people of all ages and physical conditions, as there are no risks or side effects.

How exactly are hypnotherapy treatments for IBS conducted? You have two options: in-person sessions with a hypnotherapist in your area, or use of the self-hypnosis *IBS Audio Program*.

## First option...

The first option requires finding a qualified hypnotherapist and undergoing a series of sessions in his or her office. The therapist should discuss your IBS symptoms with you and what you hope to achieve in terms of reduction. You will then lie down in a comfortable position and the therapist will use one of several techniques to induce a state of hypnosis. Once you enter this state you should feel deeply relaxed, and you will be asked to stop thinking consciously. As stress, worries, pain, and negative thoughts are cleared from your mind you will focus with intense concentration on the instructions the therapist gives you. The suggestions you're offered may use imagery or other creative thinking to help your symptoms diminish or disappear once you've returned to a normal waking state.

To achieve results, a patient needs self-motivation, repetition, and believable suggestions.[54] For IBS sufferers, the first requirement is practically a moot point. No one is more likely to want an improvement in your health than you, as you're the one suffering from the symptoms. Having this clear intention and motivation for change will help the hypnotic suggestions take hold in your subconscious and manifest successful outcomes in your daily life.

The suggestions must be reinforced by repetition. Typically, hypnotherapy sessions need to be repeated on a regular basis until you notice an improvement. Your therapist may also give you a tape of your session

---

[54] Dr. Thomas D. Yarnell, Ph.D., Clinical Psychologist.

to listen to on the days you do not have an in-person session. You are trying to change a physical health problem that you've likely been struggling
with (and emotionally impacted by) for quite some time. A single hypnotherapy session or two will not be enough to overcome your IBS—it will
take a little time and dedication to therapy on your part.

The third key to successful hypnotherapy is the use of believable suggestions. If your subconscious is to accept a suggestion, your mind must
first allow that it is a real possibility. This is why it is crucial that a hypnotherapist be knowledgeable about your particular problem (IBS or otherwise), how it physically and emotionally affects you, and what consti-
tutes a realistic address of your symptoms.

The real fly in the ointment when it comes to finding a suitable hypnotherapist for IBS is that there are so few in America with experience in
this field.[55] As a result, you will need to grill any prospective therapists
with the following questions:[56]

*Q: How long have you been practicing IBS hypnotherapy in particular?*
A: A minimum of two years is necessary simply because IBS is a complex
   syndrome, and there is really no such thing as a typical IBS patient.

*Q: Can you help IBS sufferers?*
A: If they give any other answer than an unqualified, unhesitating "yes" to
   this question, get up and leave. If they say they're willing to try and
   treat IBS though they haven't in the past, get up and leave.

*Q: What is your success rate with IBS?*
A: Hypnotherapists need not only experience with treating IBS but also
   demonstrable success rates, so they should have impressive statistics
   at their fingertips. A minimum of an eighty percent reduction in symptoms among patients is to be expected. Ask how they arrived at their
   figures, whether they conduct follow-throughs with patients, and if so
   for how long.

---

[55] The United Kingdom is another story. The British Medical Association approved hypnotherapy as a valid medical treatment in 1955, and the U.K. currently approves its use in
many situations under the national health care plan. The U.K. is one of the world leaders
in using hypnotherapy specifically for IBS; some hospital gastroenterology departments
actually employ hypnotherapists to treat the condition. The U.K. also offers a list of certified IBS Hypnotherapists. Check *http://ibs-register.co.uk/therapists.htm* for detailed information.
[56] Questions courtesy of Dr. Michael Mahoney, a clinical hypnotherapist who specializes
in the treatment of IBS.

Q: *What is IBS?*

A: A qualified IBS hypnotherapist will know that IBS is a functional digestive disorder with multiple symptoms. They will know that these symptoms can vary, and they should certainly know what the symptoms are.
If they can't name a number of symptoms with ease they're simply not
familiar with the disorder, and you should find someone else.

Q: *How many sessions will it take?*

A: You need to know this to help you budget for your treatments. IBS
should improve after two sessions and be much better by five.

Some general questions to ask a prospective hypnotherapist:

Q: *Where did you train, and for how long?*

A: There are many training organizations, and some are much more credible than others. Full-time coursework for two to three years plus an
additional year of in-service training is the minimum.

Q: *How much will this cost?*

A: You may or may not have insurance coverage for treatments. If you
don't, be cautious with payments up front.

Q: *Do you receive an audiotape of the session?*

A: Progress will result more quickly if you are given an audiotape of the
session you have just taken.

Q: *Do you have letters from past clients that I can see?*

A: Most hypnotherapists who have truly helped people, particularly with
a problem as intractable as IBS, receive overwhelming gratitude from
their patients in return. At a minimum the therapist should be able to
offer you a telephone referral to past patients who are willing and
happy to discuss their treatment and results.

Q: *Do you offer a pre-session consultation?*

A: All patients are different, particularly when it comes to IBS, so this is
a necessity. It is how a therapist gathers information about you and pre-
pares a treatment aimed at your specific needs and goals.

A question the hypnotherapist should absolutely ask you: have you
been thoroughly examined and diagnosed with IBS by a medical doctor?

If they don't ask you this they're not qualified, as any hypnotherapist familiar with IBS will know that it cannot be self-diagnosed.

## *Second option...*

If you can't find a qualified IBS hypnotherapist in your area (or are daunted by the thought of even trying) there is a second, and in my opinion, even more promising option. You can follow a set of self-hypnosis tapes, the *IBS Audio Program*, developed specifically for IBS.

*"Thanks to hypnotherapy I am eighty-five percent better."*
—Shawn Eric Case, Oregon, age 41, IBS sufferer for 31 years, unresponsive to all standard medical treatments.

*"I developed IBS symptoms following a severe case of amoebic dysentery in Mexico when I was a kid. For many years I tried various prescription drugs for IBS, as well as diets and over-the-counter products. They helped sometimes and didn't at other times, but I could not get a handle on the condition and I was caught in a vicious cycle of anxiety and symptoms which were hard to figure out.*

*Now, thanks to hypnotherapy I am eighty-five percent better. About three years ago, the pain from my IBS was very severe and I alternated between constipation and diarrhea, and I was just fed up. At this time, a great thing happened to me. I tried the IBS Audio Program and was amazed at the results. First, because I got so much better, and second, because it was from the hypnotherapy and not medications. The program worked on so many levels of my condition I was amazed, but most importantly it broke that vicious, sometimes downwards cycle I was in. Not only did my symptoms improve, but I seemed to have a much better outlook in general and I was also getting somewhere with my IBS. Nothing had worked before. IBS is a very complicated condition, and I believe the ways hypnosis works for IBS are complicated as well; however, looking back, the program was the easiest, non-medicated way for me to get better and the only thing I have found to date that worked and has continued working long-term. It has been two and a half years now since I finished the hypnotherapy program and I am still holding strong. I could write volumes on this, but I will just say that if you can find a clinical hypnotherapist who specializes in IBS give it a try. It worked for me, it has worked in research and it might work for you."*

The *IBS Audio Program* was developed through ten years of ongoing IBS research by Michael Mahoney, one of the United Kingdom's leading clinical hypnotherapists. Mahoney has over thirteen years experience as a hypnotherapist, now specializes in treating IBS patients, and is regularly referred patients by gastroenterologists and family care physicians.[57] He is an associate member of the Primary Care Society for Gastroenterology, a worldwide organization.

The IBS hypnotherapy program follows a scheduled one hundred–day treatment period and is conducted on your own time in your own home. The program is successful for over eighty percent of the patients who use it, and the reduction in symptoms and their severity averages between eighty and ninety percent for these users. It's interesting to note the significant difference in success rates for the IBS-specific hypnotherapy tapes versus general hypnotherapy tapes. In contrast to Mahoney's eighty to ninety percent success rate, general hypnotherapy tapes featuring standard relaxation techniques and visualization exercises have only produced an average fifty-seven percent improvement rate for IBS patients.[58] While any improvement is certainly better than none at all, it's clear that the benefits are far greater from a hypnotherapy program specifically developed for and aimed at IBS.

Most impressively, Mahoney's statistics arise from studies with patients who were given no relief whatsoever from conventional medical therapy— people who were, in fact, referred by gastroenterologists who had exhausted all other potential avenues of help. The incomparable success rates for the tapes are likely due to Mahoney's in-depth study and understanding of both IBS and hypnotherapy, which results in reducing anxiety, stress, and fears directly related to IBS attacks, and increasing patient confidence, self esteem, and management of IBS-specific symptoms.

---

[57] Michael Mahoney has been in hypnotherapy practice since 1987 and is affiliated with the Guardian Medical Centre in Warrington, Cheshire, England. Guardian Medical Centre is a purpose-built five partner NHS (National Health Service) training practice. In addition to training doctors and providing doctors' services, the medical center houses an operating theatre, community nurses, and other medical professionals.
[58] Mahoney, Dr. Michael. "Audiotape Hypnotherapy Treats Irritable Bowel." *Medical Tribune* 40, no. 11 (1999):13.

The IBS method of hypnotherapy developed by Mahoney is gut-specific, and termed "ongoing progressive session induction." This method was created upon the basis that as a patient responds and improves, something new must continue to happen in therapy to help the patient achieve further results. Experience has shown that if the process remains the same, the patient is more likely to become stalled at some stage of the treatment. Particularly, the sounds and words used in therapy initially, when IBS symptoms are present, can become associated with this negative state of health and mind. These same sounds and words should not continue to be used throughout the therapy because the negative associations can then become anchored onto the healing methods, which will eventually limit the progress of the patient.

The IBS method of hypnotherapy allows the patient to continue to progress throughout the entire course of treatment, and beyond. As patients learn new ways of thinking, they have more internal resources available to use in overwriting their previous negative beliefs. This then leads to further progress, more free mental resources, more progress, and the resultant reduction of IBS symptoms. Hypnotherapy works on the basis that everyone is continuously developing in one way or another, as every day involves learning, making decisions, experiencing emotions, and so on. The IBS method of treatment takes advantage of this development and encourages it by changing the sessions and mental suggestions in ways that help carry the patient continuously forward.

This approach is based on the belief that everyone throughout their lives has to keep looking for ways of moving forward, and that continuous personal development should be second nature to us all. As change is a natural part of life, we should view it as an opportunity and not a threat. The IBS method reduces the subconscious negative perceptions of change, allowing the embrace of new thoughts and beliefs, with the resultant improvement in IBS symptoms. Typically patients begin to feel much better as a result of changes in the way they think, their outlook on life, and its events, though rarely can someone pinpoint the precise moment improvements begin. These results stem from the subconscious mind, which controls the digestive system, very gently beginning to realize that the thought patterns of IBS are no longer needed. The subconscious reminds the individual as a whole that they existed very well, thank you, without IBS, and can do so again.

The audio program is complex in its makeup, but quite seamless and simple for the patient as the learning process is made easy through the use of enjoyable imagery and suggestions. The therapy itself allows changes, both physical and emotional, to occur without difficulty. Mahoney believes that just dealing with the symptoms of IBS is not enough, that the individual must learn to rebuild internal energy. Many people with IBS feel drained emotionally by the stress of living with the disorder, and the resultant crises and responsibilities in their lives continually deplete their inner emotional strength and reserves, often leading to anxiety or even depression. Before a patient can begin the process of working through their IBS, they frequently need an emotional "top-up" of these inner reserves.

In essence, they need their emotional batteries charged, as they have likely endured years of unstoppable pain and discomfort, of being told by various medical professionals that there is nothing that can be done, and intrusive or painful examinations and tests. In addition, family and work relationships may have been strained or eroded by living with an incurable illness, social and love lives may have dwindled to non-existence, and confidence and self-esteem may be at low ebb. With all of these additional stress factors the ability to put IBS in perspective is drastically reduced. If a patient begins therapy at this point, he or she will be completely unprepared for the process and unable to act upon the instructions, and failure is likely if not certain. Mahoney's program takes these IBS-specific circumstances into account, and tailors the hypnotherapy tapes to increase confidence and self-esteem first, in order to allow the patient to begin a journey of physical and emotional improvement and management. Then begins the change in their thoughts, the exchange of negative beliefs and feelings for positive ones, and the ability to move away from the symptoms and thoughts of IBS and forward toward a life without the disorder. Mahoney believes that this IBS-specific method of hypnotherapy is the best, and his patient trial results support this.

The *IBS Audio Program* itself is structured over a one hundred day period, with a listening schedule for each day (including twenty days off). The program consists of three double-sided audio cassettes or CDs, which contain an introduction and five different hypnotherapy sessions, each building on the preceding one. Sessions vary in duration but average twenty-five to thirty-five minutes. The program also includes a progress log/symptom checklist. All that is required for participation is to find a set time each day when you can listen quietly and be undisturbed. Simply fit your listening time into your daily schedule at your own convenience.

The introductory and five discrete sessions are as follows:

## INTRODUCTION

- ○ Provides detailed information about hypnotherapy, the specific process being used for the audio treatments, and information about IBS.
- ○ Acknowledges the physical and psychological combination that characterizes IBS pathology, triggers, and symptoms.
- ○ Aims to treat both IBS and the problems in a person's life that have resulted from IBS, including anxiety, social fears, depression, fatigue, and worry.
- ○ Sets a stopping point for the emotional drain of IBS; from this point on IBS symptoms will not worsen but will improve. Subconscious begins to be affected and physical changes will follow.
- ○ Emphasis on the safe, gentle, non-invasive aspects of therapy and its record as a safe form of treatment for many conditions for many years.

## FIRST SESSION

- ○ The foundation session. Allows listeners to take the time to reduce their stresses and apprehensions, to become familiar with the hypnotherapy process, and to learn that they are in control at all times.
- ○ Offers a gentle introduction to reduce anxieties and emphasize calming thoughts, thus reducing the negative thought patterns which trigger IBS physical responses.
- ○ Helps manage IBS symptoms and let users begin to understand the benefits of allowing both mind and body to work together towards the goal.

## SECOND SESSION

- ○ Begins to address the subconscious and conscious thoughts which can trigger IBS symptoms.
- ○ Teaches users, through creative imagery, to exercise control over these thoughts.

○ Uses the power of suggestion to enable listeners to learn to control the speed of peristaltic waves of the GI tract, leading to normal bowel movements.

○ Uses the mind to regulate the body.

## Third Session

○ Uses visualization to control the entire digestive process, from start to finish.

○ Begins to allow user to take control and mentally search for areas within the GI tract where there is IBS pain or discomfort, and then reduce these symptoms while continuing to use positive thoughts.

○ Negative thoughts should be decreasing and replaced by positive thoughts, which will help develop new coping strategies.

## Fourth Session

○ Uses metaphor to help view the journey through IBS as a trip that is nearing an end.

○ Acknowledges struggles of the past, the many steps the journey has required, and that while there may be a step back occasionally the progression forward will remain.

○ Acknowledges old thought patterns and allows them to be released; enhances positive thought patterns to achieve continued improvement.

○ Emphasizes that while memories of old thought patterns may remain, we don't live in the past. We live in the moment. From this moment on IBS will steadily improve, a sense of order has been reached, and progress will now continue on its own.

## Fifth Session

○ Encapsulates positive moments from the five previous sections.

○ Reaffirms the effects of the program.

○ Listeners are encouraged to review this session occasionally after the program ends to optimize their positive changes.

Of the five sessions, some are listened to once while others are repeated a dozen times. Content and order are both important. The program gives people the structure necessary to allow a progression to the end of IBS in their lives, with the final result of the reintroduction of both previously forbidden foods and stressful activities. These factors are meant to be reintroduced into patients' lives in a controlled and structured way, with a subconscious and conscious mindset that prevents the suffering of physical problems from these formerly attack-inducing elements. After the program is concluded, patients are encouraged to listen to the final tape for an additional period of time to ensure the learned processes are embedded into their subconscious.

The story of how Michael Mahoney developed the *IBS Audio Program*, and thus came to specialize in IBS hypnotherapy, is an interesting one. In 1991 he saw his first IBS patients, a condition he had at that time heard of but was not familiar with. He was quite distressed that his patients were being offered no help from the medical profession to alleviate their wide range of symptoms. They had in fact been termed "heart-sinks" by their gastroenterologists. Why? Because the doctors' hearts would sink whenever these patients returned for yet another appointment with no improvement in their condition.

Mahoney spent nearly two years researching IBS and developed a personal passion for helping the patients he was seeing, as they were truly suffering (and their loved ones were suffering indirectly as well). He wrote specific IBS hypnotherapy processes for their treatment, incorporating ongoing feedback from the patients, telling them up-front that this was a new area of practice for him and that he honestly had no idea what they could expect in terms of results. He did not charge any of the patients, and funded the initial research study of their treatment and follow-ups out of his own pocket. In spite of the fact that this was a novice attempt at IBS hypnotherapy, the success rate for his first round of patients was eighty percent.[59]

---

[59] This success rate was based on reduction of symptom severity, and the frequency of symptom presentation (how often symptoms occur). Pain, diarrhea, constipation, bloating, and other symptoms were quantified by the patients and individually measured, as was the perceived improvement in overall quality of life. Patients were asked to mark as a percentage the improvement they felt during the program period, immediately after the program had finished, and to commit to three follow-up periods of assessment at twelve months, twenty-four months, and thirty-six months after therapy ended. The treatment group included eleven females and four males; average age thirty-four.

For females: Average frequency of symptom presentation: 3.4 times daily. Average length of time IBS symptoms present: 8.63 years. Average length of time on medications: 5.5 years. Average reduction in medications over group: 96%.

For males: Average frequency of symptom presentation: 2.5 times daily. Average length of time IBS symptoms present: 4.75 years. Average length of time on medications: 3.8 years. Average reduction in medications: 94%. (1991 patient trials, per Michael Mahoney author interviews and private documents, February-April 2001).

Mahoney had by now realized that IBS hypnotherapy was the area in which he wanted to specialize. He continued to research the disorder, gaining an in-depth understanding of the physical condition and its multiple symptoms. He also realized the importance of the possible psychological effects of these symptoms, which could result in reduced self-confidence and self-esteem, increased stress and anxiety levels, and sometimes depression. His IBS-specific hypnotherapy processes and delivery methods were continuously refined to incorporate further patient feedback, with the constant goal of improving success rates.

After several years of IBS practice, the dramatic reduction in symptom severity and frequency of Mahoney's patients became well-known locally, and he began receiving numerous referrals from gastroenterologists as well as family physicians. In 1996 he was asked to participate in a medical research study of IBS hypnotherapy funded by the U.K. National Health Service through a gastroenterology practice at his Local Primary Care Medical Centre, to be monitored and audited by the local Health Authority Audit Commission. For this project, twenty patients were screened by the gastroenterologists and presented various symptoms of IBS. All patients were long-term sufferers, had undergone all medical-diagnostic tests, and had taken prescription medications without attaining significant relief from their symptoms. Each patient underwent Mahoney's introductory and five subsequent hypnotherapy sessions. The patients were split into groups, and the hypnotherapy sessions for all groups were staggered over twelve months. At the end of the project, feedback sheets from the patients indicated an overall reduction of eighty percent in symptom severity and frequency of presentation.

The success of this independent research project, to Mahoney's delight, confirmed his informal findings from earlier patient treatments in private practice. However, he now had additional patient feedback to work with, and this allowed him to further refine various aspects of the hypnotherapy delivery methods and processes.

By this point, Mahoney was receiving referrals from doctors, gastroenterologists, and other medical professionals for patients who lived over one hundred miles away. While it was gratifying to have his work recognized, it was also apparent that it was not practical for people to have to travel so far to find a hypnotherapist who understood IBS and could address the condition. At this time, early 1997, Mahoney set up the

U.K. Register of IBS Therapists and began delivering structured, comprehensive IBS-specific workshops to formally trained and experienced hypnotherapists. The IBS Register is a nonprofit organization that continues to be administered by Mahoney, and currently lists over eighty members in England and Ireland.

By mid 1997, Mahoney was also migrating new processes, information, and delivery methods for IBS hypnotherapy onto audiotapes—eventually, these would become the *IBS Audio Program*. He then began a new research study, again using out-of-pocket funds, to monitor patients using the audiotapes both during the program and for the next three subsequent years. The final results of this study are due in 2001 and are intended for independent publication so that they may be subject to peer review and analysis. Ongoing results from the study indicate a greater reduction in symptom presentation and frequency than obtained from the previous hypnotherapy methods—in fact, the success rate is close to or exceeding ninety percent for all symptoms and patients.[60]

By early 1998, it was clear to Mahoney that the audio program was offering significant help to people with IBS.[61] He attempted to gain funding for further research, development, and distribution of the IBS-hypnotherapy program, writing to every pharmaceutical company in the U.K. that manufactured prescription IBS medications. Only two companies bothered to respond, and both declined. He then made the same request to eighteen U.K. companies that produced over-the-counter IBS product. None replied. He then tried to contact the purchasing managers of various health care organizations, and received just one response—a refusal.

At this point, Mahoney determined to proceed with further development of the *IBS Audio Program* and continue the ongoing research trials with his own funds; he re-mortgaged his family home to do so, and began advertising the program.

---

[60] Patient trial results are recorded from: End of therapy program in February 1998; Year 1 following the program, February 1999; Year 2 February 2000; and Year 3 February 2001. Final study results and presentation are currently being readied for publication, but initial analysis shows a success rate close to or exceeding ninety percent for all symptoms and patients. (Per Michael Mahoney author interviews and private documents, February-April 2001).

[61] In fact, the success rate of the audio program was a mere 3.5% less than the success rate of in-person IBS hypnotherapy by Mahoney himself. (Per Michael Mahoney author interviews and private documents, February-April 2001).

In June 1999, he launched the program at the Your Health Show in London, began internet advertising, and came into contact with American and Canadian IBS Web sites and support boards. His program began to receive glowing reviews from users around the world, and IBS patients who had achieved dramatic results from the program offered their support and assistance in making the hypnotherapy tapes known to others. As of early 2001, Mahoney had been able to pay off his mortgage and is now putting new income from the program back into further research and development.[62]

I've spoken to Michael Mahoney extensively about the *IBS Audio Program*, how he developed it, the results he's achieved, and the struggles he faced along the way. The path he traveled from idea to end product was long, arduous, and quite costly to him personally, in terms of both finances and time. I related very well to his story as in many ways it closely mirrored my own experience with the *Eating for IBS* diet and cookbook. The one thing that had kept me going in the face of uninterested and uncaring medical authorities was the incredibly heartfelt and poignant letters I received from IBS sufferers, thanking me for the information and help which had often quite literally given them their lives back. When I asked Michael Mahoney what had kept him going, he told the exact same tale. It was the gratitude of his patients, as well as that of their loved ones, that enabled him to pursue an avenue at great personal expense, with little chance for much personal gain. He has said that, "those first patients and their desperation will be remembered for the rest of my life." When he began developing his program, there was little help or hope for sufferers. His commitment was driven by the need to help these people, as they had literally nowhere else to turn. His determination was simply steeled when he met with silence, refusals, and even insults from officials whose assistance he sought. Nothing else mattered once he'd decided on his own that his IBS patients were worth fighting for—the sheer gratitude he received from them had guaranteed that.

---

[62] He began a new audio program trial in November 2000 with forty-five patients, using new hypnotherapy processes. Patients are showing a quicker reduction in both severity of symptoms and frequency of presentation, and exhibit greater improvement from premenstrual related symptoms, than in previous audio program trials. Final results are due October 2001, with publication anticipated for 2002–2003. (Per Michael Mahoney author interviews and private documents, February–April 2001).

Today, as the *IBS Audio Program* gains notice as one of the most successful avenues of treatment, Mahoney is finally receiving the acknowledgment his work deserves. While he is understandably thrilled, he is plainly happier to just know that he has made a difference in the lives of many sufferers, and the lives of their families and friends as well. While he does not personally struggle with IBS, it is fair to say that he has lived with it for many years, and that he well understands the frustration, fear, and pain the disorder causes. He also knows firsthand the anger that stems from being treated dismissively by health professionals who deny the serious impact of IBS, and who simply refuse to listen to those who offer new avenues of help.

On a personal note, I believe the audio hypnotherapy program has achieved dramatic success in controlling IBS symptoms matched only by the *Eating for IBS* diet. Nothing else I have seen even comes close. There are some solid medical reasons why this would be true, and as the positive results from hypnotherapy gain recognition I hope the treatment becomes a standard option presented to patients by their physicians. I have actually been so impressed by the statistical results from hypnotherapy and the anecdotes of patients, as well as by the personal story behind Michael Mahoney's work, that I am planning to begin this treatment myself using the *IBS Audio Program*. Although I suffer only a few attacks each year at this point, they are severe and typically strike out of nowhere, and I would give dearly to be free of them entirely. I've got my fingers crossed that hypnotherapy will work as well for me as it has for so many others. If you too are interested in trying hypnotherapy (and honestly, you have little to lose and much to gain), check the resources below.

As an aside, I have no financial stake in any of these products, and nothing whatsoever to personally gain by recommending them.

## *Resources*

**IBS Hypnotherapy Tapes by Michael Mahoney**
The United Kingdom Register of IBS Therapists
P.O. Box 57, Warrington, WA5 1FG, England
Phone: 01925-629899
*www.ibsaudioprogram.com*
Cost: $98 U.S.
Delivery: approximately ten days

## Local hypnotherapists

Legally, anyone can practice hypnotherapy without training or a license. So if you wish to see a hypnotherapist in your area for personal sessions, it's important to make sure you find a professional. Most are physicians or psychologists with thorough training in hypnotherapy. It is also crucial that your therapist have experience with treating IBS specifically, and it won't hurt to just spend a little time with the practitioner you're considering to determine whether you have good personal rapport. The average cost of a hypnotherapy session ranges from sixty to one hundred twenty dollars and upwards. To find a therapist, you can ask your gastroenterologist or family physician for a reference, or contact one of these organizations:

**American Council of Hypnotist Examiners**
700 S. Central Ave.
Glendale, CA 91204
Phone: 818-242-5378
*www.sonic.net/hypno/ache.html*

**The American Institute of Hypnotherapy**
1805 East Garryn Ave., Suite 100
Santa Ana, CA 92705
Phone: 714-261-6400

*The American Society of Clinical Hypnosis*
2200 East Devon Ave., Suite 291
Des Plaines, IL 60018
Phone: 708-297-3317
*www.asch.net*

**International Medical and Dental Hypnotherapy Association**
International Headquarters
4110 Edgeland, Suite 800
Royal Oak, MI 48073-2285
Phone: 248-549-5594 (800-257-5467 outside Michigan)
*www.infinityinst.com*

**Milton H. Erickson Foundation**
3606 North 24 Street
Phoenix, AZ 85016
Phone: 602-956-6196
*www.erickson-foundation.org*

**The National Guild of Hypnotists**
P.O. Box 308
Merrimack, NH 03054-0308
Phone: 603-429-9438
*www.ngh.net*

## IN A SENTENCE:

*Alternative therapies, particularly acupuncture and hypnotherapy, can be specifically tailored to address IBS symptoms, and can reduce the frequency, severity, and duration of attacks with minimal risk of side effects.*

# MILESTONE

By the end of your first week you've taken the first crucial steps to regaining your health as quickly as possible, as you have now:

○ VERIFIED YOUR DIAGNOSIS

○ LEARNED THE PHYSIOLOGY OF IBS

○ IMPLEMENTED THE FIVE KEY STRATEGIES FOR CONTROLLING YOUR SYMPTOMS

*task list*

1. CLEAN OUT YOUR PANTRY AND GIVE AWAY THOSE TRIGGER FOODS.

2. MAKE A GROCERY LIST OF YOUR NEW STAPLES.

3. GO SHOPPING AND RE-STOCK YOUR KITCHEN WITH SAFE FOODS (AND ANY NECESSARY COOKING EQUIPMENT).

4. START PLANNING DAILY MENUS.

5. ADAPT RECIPES AND BEGIN TO COOK FOR IBS.

# Eating Enjoyably at Home

**AFTER A** week of eating safely for IBS, your digestion should have stabilized, and as you enter your second week you can now expand your diet from the soluble fiber foods you've been limited to. You will still, *always*, need to base each snack and meal on soluble fiber, and follow the ten commandments of eating safely, but you should now be ready to begin stocking your kitchen, cooking, and eating a wider variety of great foods at home. This will require cleaning out your pantry, making lots of lists, shopping for a supply of safe staples, and re-stocking your kitchen. Further down the road in Month 11 we'll take a trip to explore places like Asian or Indian markets and whole food/health food grocery stores to expand your home cooking options even further.

Once all this prep work is done you'll be ready to plan your daily menus, adapt recipes, and start cooking. The entire process should be a lot of fun, so I hope you're looking forward to it. After all, not only can you now expect to eat without fear of an attack, you also have a lifetime of fabulous meals to look forward to.

## *Empty your pantry*

You're going to fill your kitchen with lots of new safe staples, but first you need to make room for them in your pantry, freezer, and fridge. This will probably be pretty easy once you toss out all the trigger foods that are occupying space right now. So give away the ice cream, Cool Whip, potato chips, cheese, salad dressings, milk, ground beef, steak, bologna, mayonnaise, candy bars, and any other meat, dairy, or high-fat culprits. Take a moment of silence for their departure from your life, and permit yourself a deep sigh of regret if you must, but realize that what you're really giving up here is the dread of attacks and the agony of enduring them. Good health can still be delicious—I promise.

Now, arm yourself with pen and paper and make a list of all the staples you'll be buying:

> white bread such as French or sourdough (extra loaves for the freezer)[1]
> pasta (no egg noodles)
> rice noodles (in the Asian foods section)
> rice (short or long grain, jasmine, basmati, rose, any white variety will do, even Minute!)
> flour tortillas (freeze 'em)
> potatoes (white and sweet) and other root vegetables
> oatmeal

---

[1] Remember, it's not wheat flour that's a trigger, it's *whole wheat* flour. White breads are great, safe staples.

Cream of Rice

Rice Chex or Corn Chex

baked corn chips (like Tostitos)

baked potato chips (Lays)

pretzels

cooking oil spray (like Pam)

organic eggs (buy extra—you'll only be using the whites—or get pow-
    dered whites)

bananas, mangoes, and unsweetened applesauce (the few safe fruits)

amazake rice drinks (if you can find them—they're usually only at
    health food stores)

soy, rice, or oat milk (fat-free—try several brands and choose a
    favorite)

peppermint or other IBS herbal tea, or bulk herbs to brew (see
    Month 2 for choices)

Metamucil, Citrucel, and/or Fibercon (soluble fiber supplements—
    *not* laxatives—discussed in detail in Month 2)

Next stop, your biggest and best local food market. Ready, set, shop!
Your mission is to fill your cart and your kitchen with soluble fiber staples,
so you're never at a loss for the basis of a meal or snack. At no time in your
future will you ever again stand in the middle of your kitchen with the
refrigerator and cupboard doors wide open, wondering what on earth you
can eat. From this day forward you will have safe staples any time you
need them, and it's hard to underestimate the peace of mind this will
bring. Somehow just knowing that you have the right foods on hand at all
times can mean so much less worry about your diet, you will actually save
yourself some attacks from the elimination of stress you used to endure
while wondering how and what to eat.

While you're shopping, supplement your staples by adding:

fresh seafood of any kind[2]
skinless chicken/turkey breasts or shaved deli chicken/turkey breasts
    (try to buy organic)
tofu
dried or canned beans of any kind (you'll be using them carefully,
    with soluble fiber)
lentils (ditto)
your favorite fresh fruits and vegetables (ditto again, and try to buy
    organic)
almonds, pecans, or walnuts (you'll be grinding them and adding
    them to soluble fiber)
fat-free veggie broth powder
canola and olive oil (which you'll use very sparingly and with soluble
    fiber)

These foods will round out your meals and snacks for good health and great taste, and are all safe when eaten properly and added to your soluble fiber staples.

If you've got some space left in that grocery cart, you can consider adding some safe splurge foods:

angel food cake mix (we all need a treat sometimes,
    and this is super-safe)
cocoa powder (for safe baking)
sorbets
soy or rice milk ice creams (make sure they're low-fat)
Corn Pops or Honeycomb cereals (a great, sweet, and stabilizing
    snack right out of the box)
fortune cookies
peppermint hard candies

---

[2] Interestingly, even fatty fish such as tuna and salmon don't seem to typically cause any problems for IBS. This may be because they contain omega-3 and omega-6 essential fatty acids, which can have an inflammation-reducing effect on the colon.

---

### Why Buy Organic?

**ALTHOUGH THERE** haven't been any studies on the effects of organic versus non-organic poultry, eggs, and produce on people with IBS, many sufferers feel that their GI tracts are simply more sensitive to all chemicals, drugs, and preservatives in general. Since there is certainly no downside to buying organic foods, and as an upside there is always the chance that you are preventing exposure to triggers, you may want to just go organic as a matter of course.

---

You'll notice that these are all sweet treats, as the great thing about eating for IBS is that there is at least one typically safe junk food—refined sugar. Not desserts as a rule, mind you, because those are almost always very high-fat and often dairy-based as well. But sugar in the form of sucrose, like your average baking white and brown sugars, is not a GI stimulant or irritant (as opposed to fructose), and it contains no fat or insoluble fiber. This means that you have the option of eating sweets without worry if they fall within the IBS dietary guidelines,[3] and as long as you don't overindulge (sugar is most definitely not a health food).

Once you've finished your grocery shopping, you might need to make a trip to a local cooking supply shop and add to your kitchen a set of nonstick skillets, baking pans, and rubber spatulas/wooden spoons to use with them. Nonstick pans are really essential for cooking for IBS, as they easily allow you to use the bare minimum of cooking oil spray, or even no oil at all.

Okay, you're back home, you've restocked your kitchen, and your pantry, freezer, and fridge are bursting with safe staples…now what?

---

[3] See *Eating for IBS* (Marlowe & Company, 2000), by Heather Van Vorous, for one hundred seventy-five safe recipes for IBS, including a dessert chapter.

*living*

# Let's Get Cooking!

**ONE OF** the best ways for people to manage their IBS through diet is to know ahead of time exactly what (and even when) they'll be eating. You might want to make a list the night before of all your meals and snacks for the next day. The idea here is simple peace of mind. If you know that you will be eating safely because you already have the food on hand and prepared, you are assured that your diet will be a source of stability instead of trouble.

Try making a daily menu plan for this whole week. I've included two separate three-day sample menus for people who either love or hate to cook, and they both give very generous quantities and clear guidelines you can follow. You can also mix and match the days to arrive at a full week's worth of menus, or you can create your own meals from scratch right from the start if you're feeling more ambitious.

# Quick Tips for Adapting Recipes to the IBS Kitchen

○ Replace all dairy milk with soy, rice, or oat milk (check labels to make sure no oil has been added, and use unsweetened varieties for savory recipes).

○ To replace buttermilk, sour 1 cup soy milk with 1 teaspoon–1 tablespoon vinegar. (This is called clabbering.)

○ Replace sour cream, cream cheese, ice cream, cheese, and all other dairy products with soy, rice, or almond substitutes (widely available at health food stores).

○ Replace ground meat and eliminate the cooking oil in recipes (such as chili or sloppy Joes) by using TVP, a textured soy product available at health food stores.

○ Replace bacon with "Fakin' Bacon," a smoked tempeh (soy) product at health food stores (you won't believe the terrific smoky flavor this lends to soups and dips).

○ Replace regular mayonnaise and salad dressings with fat-free versions (spike them with a little fresh lemon juice and some minced fresh herbs for more flavor).

○ Substitute cocoa powder for solid chocolate when baking. (Not only is cocoa powder almost fat-free, but the caffeine in cocoa beans is tied to the fat, which means cocoa powder is also very low in caffeine.)

○ Replace most of the oil in baked goods with applesauce or other fruit purées.

○ Make all pies with low-fat graham crusts instead of pastry crusts.

○ Use a little blended silken tofu to thicken sauces and soups.

○ Use cooked peeled potatoes, cubed white bread, or firm tofu as a low-fat and high soluble fiber base for creamy dips, sauces, and spreads (just whirl with liquids and seasonings in a food processor).

○ Purée vegetable and bean or lentil soups until smooth to minimize their insoluble fiber, and to thicken them without roux (a mixture of oil and flour).

○ Replace each whole egg with two egg whites.

○ Replace most oil in sauces and soups with veggie broth (available at health food stores).

○ Instead of pan- or deep-frying, make foods brown and crispy by frying with cooking oil spray in a nonstick skillet.

○ Remember that fat carries flavor, so when you reduce the fat in a recipe you should increase the herbs and spices.

○ When baking, use generous quantities of vanilla and other extracts, as well as spices such as cinnamon and nutmeg, to heighten the richness and sweetness.

○ Never butter or oil pans for baking—just spray lightly with cooking oil.

If you'd like to start modifying your own recipes, just follow the general rules you've learned for carefully incorporating insoluble fiber into the soluble fiber staples, minimizing all fats, substituting soy or rice products for dairy, using two egg whites to replace a whole egg, and so on. The vast majority of recipes, from homestyle cooking to ethnic foods to rich desserts, can all be pretty easily adapted to the IBS kitchen with delicious results. You'll quickly learn through trial and error which recipes are most easily modified and you'll soon have your own collection of personal IBS recipes that are safe and scrumptious. You may well find that friends and family don't even realize you've been tinkering with their tried-and-true favorites, as many recipes will still taste exactly the same. I learned years ago to simply not tell people that my cooking was tailored for my own health needs. I just served them good food and it never occurred to them that there was something missing (like fat, or meat, or dairy) because the end result still tasted great. What people don't know....

## Three-Day Sample Menu with Quick and Easy Recipes for People who Love to Cook

I've included a wide variety of recipes here. Each showcases at least one feature of the simple modifications that allow you to cook and eat safely for IBS—without sacrificing an ounce of flavor. Several of the recipes demonstrate how a high soluble fiber base, (whether rice, pasta, oatmeal, white bread, cornmeal, or white flour) allows you to incorporate the insoluble fiber of fresh vegetables and fruits by cooking and finely chopping or blending them. Other recipes use legumes and nuts similarly added to soluble fiber, and finely ground or puréed for safety. Several recipes replace dairy products with soy substitutes for terrific results, and breakfast as well as baked goods show just how easy it is to use only egg whites instead of whole eggs. The delicious breads and desserts demonstrate how little oil actually needs to be included in baking, by turning to cocoa powder instead of high-fat solid chocolate and using applesauce for the rich, moist texture typically obtained with butter. I've tried to include some exciting ethnic recipes as well, to make the point that safe does not mean boring or bland, and to give you a starting point for expanding your cooking repertoire into more adventurous meals. One recipe in particular showcases the surprising element of hot and spicy flavors, which are rendered safe by the low-fat, high soluble fiber foundation of the meal. Enjoy!

## DAY 1.

BREAKFAST   Wild mushroom and thyme scrambled eggs on sourdough toast. Small banana. Peppermint (or other herbal) tea.

SNACK   Maple oat bread. Peppermint (or other herbal) tea.

LUNCH   Red lentil soup with cumin-caraway toast. Small mango.

SNACK   Handful of baked corn chips. Peppermint (or other herbal) tea.

DINNER   Asparagus and lemon pasta. French bread. Chocolate cherry pound cake.

## DAY 2.

BREAKFAST   Cinnamon peach oatmeal. Peppermint (or other herbal) tea.

SNACK   Apple spice walnut bread. Peppermint (or other herbal) tea.

LUNCH   Bagel sandwich with shaved deli chicken breast, maple-dijon mustard, cucumber, basil leaves, avocado, and tomatoes. Handful of pretzels. Small pear.

SNACK   Maple oat bread and small banana or peeled pear. Glass vanilla soy milk.

DINNER   Mexican mango shrimp with rice. Blueberry pecan cake.

## DAY 3.

BREAKFAST   Cornmeal cream cheese pancakes with cranberry-apricot syrup. Small banana. Peppermint (or other herbal) tea.

SNACK   Apple spice walnut bread. Peppermint (or other herbal) tea.

LUNCH   Sourdough sandwich with crab, mango chutney, tofu cream cheese, cucumbers, and watercress. Small handful fresh strawberries.

SNACK   Handful of pretzels or rice cake. Peppermint (or other herbal) tea.

DINNER   Roasted miso salmon with rice. Steamed sweet potatoes and zucchini. Blueberry pecan cake.

# wild mushroom and thyme scrambled eggs on sourdough toast

**SCRAMBLED EGGS** are so easy to make safe for IBS—just omit the yolks and use only whites, and fry with cooking spray in a nonstick skillet. Adding sautéed wild mushrooms makes for a truly special breakfast dish, and the sourdough toast gives a nice soluble fiber foundation. The touch of sherry demonstrates how small amounts of alcohol can be safely incorporated into recipes for heightened flavor.

**Makes 1 serving (easily doubled or tripled)**

2 organic egg whites

dash salt

½ tablespoon fresh thyme, or ½ teaspoon dried

⅔ cup assorted wild mushrooms (oyster, portobello, shitake, etc.), cleaned and chopped

1 garlic clove, minced

1 teaspoon–1 tablespoon sherry (or cooking sherry), to taste

1 large slice sourdough bread, toasted

In a small bowl, whisk together egg whites with thyme and salt. Set aside. In a small nonstick skillet sprayed with cooking oil, sauté the mushrooms and garlic over medium heat until tender, and liquid from mushrooms has evaporated. Add egg mixture and sherry and cook, stirring, over medium heat until egg has cooked through. Spoon over toast and serve.

# maple oat bread

**THIS BREAD** is a delicious, terrific staple to bake in large batches so you have extra loaves to freeze. The oatmeal and flour give a high soluble fiber content, while the soured soy milk tenderizes the dough in place of the traditional buttermilk. Either pecans or cranberries are a lovely touch that perfectly complements the maple richness of this bread.

### Makes 1 9 x 5" loaf, doubles easily

1¾ cups all-purpose unbleached white flour

1 teaspoon baking powder

½ teaspoon baking soda

½ teaspoon salt

2 organic egg whites

¼ cup canola oil

½ cup maple syrup

3 tablespoon packed brown sugar

1½ cups soy milk blended with 1 tablespoon vinegar

1 cup regular or quick rolled oats

⅓ cup finely chopped pecans *or* chopped dried cranberries (optional)

Preheat oven to 350°F. Lightly spray a 9 x 5" loaf pan with cooking oil. In a large bowl, sift the flour, baking powder, baking soda, and salt. Whisk together until blended. In a medium bowl whisk the egg whites with the oil until smooth. Whisk in the maple syrup, brown sugar, and soured soy milk. Stir in the oats. (Add pecans or dried cranberries.)

Add wet ingredients to dry and stir with a wooden spoon until just combined. Pour into pan, smooth top, and bake until golden brown and a tester inserted into center of loaf comes out clean, about 1 hour. Cool on rack in pan for 10 minutes, then turn out of pan onto rack and cool completely before slicing. Freezes beautifully.

# red lentil soup with cumin-caraway toasts

**HERE'S A** hearty, throw-together, Middle Eastern-style soup that is wonderful on autumn or winter days. Puréeing the soup minimizes the insoluble fiber of the lentil skins, while the insides of the legume offer lots of soluble fiber. Gently spiced sourdough toasts increase the soluble fiber even more, and add a tasty crunch as well.

**Makes 8–10 servings**

*Soup:*

2½ cups dried red lentils (about 1 pound), picked over for stones

2 medium onions, finely chopped

5 large garlic cloves, minced

2 tablespoons olive oil

1 tablespoon ground coriander

1½ teaspoons ground cumin

2 large cinnamon sticks

½ teaspoon ground cardamom

⅛ teaspoon ground cloves

1 teaspoon ground ginger

½ teaspoon white pepper

8 cups veggie broth

1½ teaspoons salt

In a large bowl soak lentils in cold water to cover for 1 hour, then drain. In a large heavy stockpot sauté onions and garlic in oil over medium heat, stirring, until golden. Stir in spices (but not salt) and cook, stirring occasionally, about five minutes. Stir in lentils and broth and bring to a boil. Reduce heat and simmer uncovered until lentils disintegrate, stirring occasionally, about 1 hour (though the longer this soup cooks the tastier it will be). Add the salt and remove the cinnamon sticks. Purée about half the soup in a blender and return to pot. Serve with one piece of toast at bottom of each bowl, and top each bowl with second piece of toast.

*Cumin-caraway toasts:*

    2 small pieces of sourdough bread per person
    ground cumin
    ground caraway seeds
    garlic salt

Lightly mist both sides of bread with cooking oil spray. Sprinkle lightly with cumin, caraway, and garlic salt. Toast until golden brown.

# asparagus and lemon pasta

**HERE'S THE** perfect summer meal. It's light, flavorful, a beautiful gold and green, and nutritious to boot. It's also high soluble fiber and very low-fat, with most of the asparagus puréed into a rich sauce in order to minimize the insoluble fiber. You can try lots of variations of this pasta by substituting fresh peas, artichoke hearts, or other greens for the asparagus.

**Makes 4 servings**

1 lb. fresh asparagus, ends trimmed
zest of 1 fresh lemon
2 tablespoons extra-virgin olive oil
1 lb. bowtie pasta (or pasta or choice)
¼ cup soy Parmesan cheese (optional)

Cut asparagus into 1" pieces, setting aside tips. In a large stockpot cook asparagus stems in 5–6 quarts boiling water with 1 tablespoon salt until very tender (about 7–9 minutes). Transfer asparagus with a slotted spoon to a blender (do not drain pot). Cook asparagus tips in same boiling water until just tender, about 4–5 minutes. Transfer tips with slotted spoon to colander (do not drain pot).

Purée asparagus stems (not the tips) with lemon zest, olive oil, and 3/4 cup asparagus cooking water until smooth.

Cook pasta in boiling asparagus cooking water until it's still very al dente (firm to the tooth). Reserve 2 cups cooking water and drain pasta. In drained stockpot, add pasta, asparagus tips, asparagus sauce, and 1/2 cup reserved water. Cook over high heat, stirring, about 4–5 minutes until pasta is done to taste and coated with sauce, adding a little more cooking water (1/4 cup at a time) if necessary. Stir in soy Parmesan and salt and pepper to taste. Serve immediately.

# chocolate cherry pound cake

**THIS CAKE** is deep, dark, and devilishly rich with chocolate—the luscious addition of fresh cherries just sends it right over the top into pure dessert heaven. It's the perfect example of how simple kitchen wizardry—applesauce for most of the oil, cocoa powder instead of solid chocolate—can turn even the most decadent recipe into a safe low-fat, high soluble fiber indulgence.

**Makes 12 servings**

Preheat oven to 325°F. Spray a 10" nonstick bundt cake pan with cooking oil and set aside.

In a large bowl sift, then whisk together:

    2 cups all-purpose unbleached white flour
    1 cup granulated sugar
    2 teaspoons baking soda
    1/3 cup unsweetened cocoa powder (I have the best results with
        Hershey's)
    1 tablespoon cornstarch
    1/2 teaspoon salt

In a medium bowl whisk together:

    1 3/4 cups unsweetened applesauce (homemade or bottled)
    1/4 cup canola oil
    1 tablespoon vanilla extract
    1 teaspoon almond extract
    1 1/2 cups fresh cherries, pitted and diced (or 3/4 cup dried cherries, diced)

Add the wet ingredients to the dry with a few swift strokes until just blended. Pour into prepared bundt pan. Bake for 50–60 minutes, or until a tester comes out with moist crumbs. Cool on rack.

# cinnamon peach oatmeal

**HERE'S A** quick breakfast that shows just how easy it is to safely eat fresh fruit as long as it's prepared properly (peeled, diced, and cooked) and combined with soluble fiber (from the oatmeal). Just as importantly, it's absolutely delicious.

**Makes 1 serving (can be easily doubled)**

½ cup rolled oatmeal (not instant)
1 cup vanilla soy or rice milk
1 teaspoon brown sugar
½ teaspoon cinnamon
1 whole fresh peach, skinned and pitted, diced

Combine all ingredients in a microwave-safe bowl large enough to prevent boil-over, and stir well. Microwave on high for 2 minutes (or cook in saucepan over stove at medium heat) and stir. Microwave another 1–2 minutes, until oatmeal is thickened.

# apple spice walnut bread

**THIS BREAD** is simply fabulous—it will perfume your whole house as it bakes. The recipe shows how safe and easy it can be to add a little whole wheat to your cooking, as you're combining it with a very high soluble fiber base of oatmeal, white flour, and applesauce. It's this foundation that also allows you to add ground walnuts to the sweetly spiced topping.

### Makes 1 9 x 5" loaf

Preheat oven to 350°F. Spray loaf pan with cooking oil and set aside.

In a large bowl beat together with an electric mixer:

   3 tablespoons canola oil

   3 organic egg whites

   ¼ cup maple syrup

   ½ cup unsweetened applesauce (homemade or bottled)

   ½ cup soy milk mixed with 1 teaspoon vinegar

   ½ cup brown sugar, packed

   1 teaspoon maple extract

   1 teaspoon vanilla extract

Stir in:

   1 medium-tart apple, peeled, cored, and finely diced (about 1 cup)

   1 cup rolled oats (not instant)

In a large bowl sift, then whisk together:

   ¾ cup plus 2 tablespoons all-purpose unbleached white flour

   ½ cup whole wheat pastry flour

   2 teaspoons baking powder

   ½ teaspoon baking soda

   ½ teaspoon salt

   1 tablespoon cinnamon

Add the wet ingredients to the dry with a few swift strokes until blended. Pour into prepared loaf pan and smooth top. Sprinkle evenly with topping.

Bake about 1 hour, or until a tester comes out clean. Cool on rack.

*Topping:*
  2 tablespoons brown sugar
  2 tablespoons ground walnuts
  ¼ teaspoon nutmeg
  ¼ teaspoon ginger
  ¼ teaspoon cloves
  ½ teaspoon cinnamon

# mexican mango shrimp with rice

**THIS SUBTLY** sweet and earthy dish will come as a happy surprise to many people. It meets the basic low-fat, high soluble fiber requirements, but it also adds in a spicy note with the use of the Thai chili sauce, Sriracha. How can this be safe? Most spicy foods that people know from experience are dangerous (chili, tacos, sloppy Joes, etc.) aren't actually problematic due to their seasoning, but their typical high-fat, meat, and cheese content. Once you remove those trigger foods and reduce the oil, then add in a high soluble fiber base, the spices themselves can simply be treated like insoluble fiber and safely incorporated. Once again, the lesson is that the IBS diet does not require any sacrifice in flavor, but instead gives you the opportunity to expand into new tastes and cooking adventures.

### Makes 2–3 servings, easily doubled

8 oz. medium to large shrimp, shelled and deveined, tails removed

1 cup puréed fresh mango

¼ cup pepitas, toasted in a dry skillet, and ground to powder*

1–2 tablespoons Sriracha sauce**

salt to taste

1 cup cooked long grain white rice (such as jasmine or basmati)

## *for serving:*

2–3 flour tortillas

½ cup finely shredded cabbage

1 small avocado, diced

1 tablespoon minced fresh cilantro

Combine shrimp, mango, ground pepitas, Sriracha, and salt in a glass pie plate, and marinate for 30 minutes. Sauté mixture in a nonstick skillet until shrimp are just cooked through, about 3 minutes, stirring frequently. Fold in rice. Spoon mixture into tortillas and add a sprinkle of cabbage and avocado, roll up tortillas, top with cilantro, and serve.

*Pepitas are green pumpkin seeds, available at health food stores, Indian markets, or Hispanic markets. To toast them spread evenly in a dry skillet, and cook over medium-high heat, stirring constantly, until they pop and are lightly golden but not brown. Let cool and finely grind in a spice grinder, blender, or food processor.

**Sriracha is a fantastic Thai vinegar-chili sauce that is not simply hot but full of flavor. It's available at many health food stores, in the ethnic section of some grocery stores, and any Asian market.

# blueberry pecan cake

**HERE'S MY** favorite coffee cake, though it makes a delicious dessert as well. It's a good example of how finely grinding nuts can minimize their insoluble fiber, and how cooking fruit and combining it with soluble fiber (from both the flour and pecans) makes it safe. This cake is very pretty, with plump blueberries dotted among the crunchy-topped, spicy golden cake.

### Makes 14-16 servings

¾ cup pecans, finely ground

½ cup packed brown sugar

¼ teaspoon nutmeg

⅓ cup plus 3 tablespoons all-purpose unbleached white flour

6 large organic egg whites

¼ teaspoon salt

¼ cup canola oil

2 teaspoons vanilla extract

2 cups fresh or frozen blueberries (if frozen do not thaw)

½ teaspoon granulated sugar

Preheat oven to 375°F. Spray a 10" nonstick springform pan with cooking oil and set aside. In a medium bowl whisk together pecans, brown sugar, nutmeg, and flour until well combined. In a large bowl beat egg whites with salt until they just hold stiff peaks and fold in nut mixture gently but thoroughly. Fold in oil and vanilla extract, and spread batter in prepared pan.

Arrange berries evenly over batter and sprinkle with granulated sugar. Bake cake for 25–30 minutes or until a tester comes out clean. Cool on rack.

# cornmeal cream cheese pancakes with cranberry-apricot syrup

**THE PANCAKES** are a special treat for breakfast or a weekend brunch. They show how beautifully soy substitutes can replace dairy (cream cheese and milk) with delicious results. Whole eggs have been replaced by egg whites to minimize the fat content, and the soluble fiber of the flour and cornmeal make the addition of small amounts of dried fruit in the syrup perfectly tolerable.

**Makes 4 servings**

*Syrup:*
- 1 cup pure maple syrup
- ¼ cup chopped dried cranberries
- ¼ cup chopped dried apricots
- 2 teaspoons fresh lemon juice

Simmer all ingredients except lemon juice in a saucepan over medium low heat until fruits are soft, about 5 minutes. Remove from heat and stir in lemon juice.

*Pancakes:*
- ¾ cup unbleached all-purpose white flour
- ½ cup yellow cornmeal
- 1½ teaspoons baking powder
- ½ teaspoon baking soda
- 1 tablespoon brown sugar
- 2 tablespoons granulated sugar
- ½ teaspoon salt
- ⅔ cup tofu cream cheese (available at health food stores)
- 4 egg whites
- ¾ cup vanilla soy milk

In a large bowl whisk together flour, cornmeal, baking powder, baking soda, both sugars, and salt. In a medium bowl whisk together tofu cream cheese and egg whites. Gradually whisk in soy milk until smooth. Add wet ingredients to dry and whisk until just combined.

Heat a large nonstick skillet over medium heat and spray with cooking oil. Spoon large tablespoons of batter onto pan, without crowding. Cook 1–2 minutes per side, until golden and puffed. Top with syrup and serve.

# roasted miso salmon with rice

**THIS IS** an all-time favorite fish recipe of mine. The preparation and cooking couldn't be faster and easier, but you do have to allow at least one day for marinating. If you've never cooked with miso paste before you're in for a treat. It has a unique sweet-yet-salty-flavor that melds beautifully with the fish. The rice gives this meal its soluble fiber base.

### Makes 3–4 servings

1 pound 1" thick salmon fillet (black cod and Chilean sea bass work
    wonderfully too)
⅓ cup miso paste*
1 tablespoon mirin or sake*
cooked white rice for serving

If fish fillets are too thick halve them horizontally. In a small bowl gradually whisk the mirin into the miso until smooth. Place fish in a large shallow baking pan lined with heavy foil, coat all sides of fish with miso sauce using a rubber spatula, and cover tightly with plastic wrap. Refrigerate for 24–48 hours.

Preheat oven to 500°F. Remove plastic wrap from fish and scrape off excess miso sauce with rubber spatula. Discard sauce. Roast salmon, uncovered, in oven until just cooked through, about 15 minutes. Transfer cooked fish to plates and serve with rice.

*Miso and mirin are both available at many grocery stores, health food stores, and Asian markets. For this recipe you can use any type of miso (white, red, yellow). Mirin is a low-alcohol, sweetened rice wine (sake) used exclusively for cooking. Any brand will do for this recipe.

## *Three-Day Sample Menu for People who Hate to Cook*

**DAY 1.**

BREAKFAST    Bowl of Rice Chex or Corn Chex with soy or rice milk and a sliced banana or mango. Peppermint tea.

SNACK    Graham crackers. Peppermint (or other herbal) tea.

LUNCH    Subway sandwich on white bread—chicken or turkey breast, mustard, tomato, small amount lettuce/onions. Lays baked potato chips. Small peeled pear.

SNACK    Handful of pretzels and dried apricots. Peppermint (or other herbal) tea.

DINNER    Chinese restaurant: mu shu veggies with extra rice, or chicken/shrimp/veggie chop suey with extra rice (ask that very little oil and no MSG be used). Fortune cookies.

**DAY 2.**

BREAKFAST    Bowl of instant oatmeal made with soy or rice milk, topped with sliced banana and mango. Or, toasted bagel with smidgen of peanut butter and marmalade. Peppermint (or other herbal) tea.

SNACK    Graham crackers. Glass vanilla soy milk.

LUNCH    Can of Campbell's tomato rice soup, or Progresso chicken noodle or vegetable soup. Fat free Saltines. Small peeled apple.

SNACK    Pretzels or rice cakes and handful dried apricots. Peppermint (or other herbal) tea.

DINNER    Italian restaurant: Dinner rolls (not whole wheat), no butter. Minestrone soup (no meat/cheese). Pasta primavera (ask for no cheese/no oil). Small green salad with fat-free vinaigrette (eat the pasta first). Small scoop fruit sorbet.

## DAY 3.

BREAKFAST    Denny's: Scrambled egg whites or egg white omelet (no cheese/butter, ask for the bare minimum of oil in the frying pan), topped with salsa. Toasted English muffins with honey or seedless jam. Small fresh fruit salad (eat it last).

SNACK    Small banana and rice cake. Peppermint (or other herbal) tea.

LUNCH    Japanese restaurant: sushi rolls, soba noodles, seaweed salad, tofu/chicken/salmon teriyaki with extra rice. Green tea.

SNACK    Graham crackers. Glass vanilla soy milk.

DINNER    Mexican restaurant: Chicken/shrimp/veggie fajitas (no cheese/sour cream), with extra flour tortillas and extra rice. Go light on the lettuce and refried beans, and ask that as little oil as possible be used in the fajitas. Peppermint (or other herbal) tea, or virgin strawberry daiquiri. (Do *not* eat the basket of corn chips—they're fried).

## IN A SENTENCE:

> *Now that your digestion has stabilized and you've learned the ten commandments of eating for IBS, it's time to clean out your pantry, shop for a supply of safe staples, re-stock your kitchen, and begin adapting recipes.*

# WEEK **3**

*learning*

## task list

1. TAKE CONTROL OF HOW YOU EAT AT WORK.

2. PLAN AHEAD FOR A MEAL AT A RESTAURANT, THEN FOLLOW THROUGH AND EAT OUT.

3. LEARN HOW TO EAT SAFELY AT A FRIEND'S HOUSE AND AT PARTIES.

# Eating Safely Away from Home

**YOU'RE BEGINNING** to establish and maintain a healthy diet at home, so let's take the next step and move on out into the world. Don't be scared, but do be careful. When you're the one who's cooking you're in total control, and you have complete knowledge of what, exactly, is in a recipe. If you're eating out things aren't so simple. When you're at work, a restaurant, a friend's house, or a party, you won't have much control over what you're eating unless you speak up, ask questions, and maybe do a little detective work as well.

## *At work*

For catered meals and snacks at work, you'll either have to avoid tak-ing risks by bringing your own food or, better still, simply make your needs known. Yes, you may become known office-wide for having IBS, but so what? At least you won't go hungry. I've found that most employers are perfectly happy to order-in lunches from restaurants I request, or (even better) order a special meal just for me. I've actually learned that this is incidentally a great way to get much better food than everyone else around me, as they are likely to be stuck with greasy fast food while I get to enjoy a lovely order of sushi rolls (which everyone else eyes with envy).

It's helpful to make friends with the office folks who do the actual ordering, and ask them to let you know in advance whenever meals will be catered so that you can try and find something suitable on the menu. I have had wonderful luck with this approach, to the extent that one com-pany I worked for simply stopped ordering food from restaurants that were difficult for me. You'd be surprised how painless it may be to be accom-modated at work in this matter—and honestly, you're also likely to find you're not the only one making special requests. There are bound to be others in the same boat, whether people with diabetes, food allergies, or simply vegetarians. So speak up and you are likely to be heard—and fed!

## *Restaurants—A scouting expedition*

The easiest way to eat safely for IBS at restaurants is to make sure you choose a good prospect in the first place. This obviously eliminates most (if not all) fast food restaurants and burger joints, but leaves you a tremendous wealth of traditional American, ethnic, and vegetarian places. It's important that, if you're eating out with friends, you speak up and make it clear that the restaurant of choice needs to serve food you can actually eat. Don't be afraid to make yourself heard. You deserve a little special consideration here, and this means that you should have veto power if everyone else wants to eat at a place that simply won't work for you. Remember that going out to eat is as much about socializing as it is about eating, so rest assured that your real friends will be happy just to be with you, regardless which particular restaurant you choose. If someone is consistently less than gracious about catering to your special dietary needs, feel free to drop them from your social circle. Anyone who doesn't consider your good health a reasonable priority is really no friend after all.

Before you venture out to eat, you may want to simply drive by all your favorite local restaurants and gather every take-out menu available. Take them home and look them over and see what your options are, and you can begin compiling a list of restaurants that you know have safe meal choices for you.

When you read the menus you're looking for low fat, high soluble fiber meals. At traditional restaurants, this might mean grilled chicken breasts or broiled seafood with a rice or pasta side dish, a pasta primavera, or a veggie fried rice. Watch out for words like "crispy," "crunchy," "creamy," and "rich," which typically signify fried or dairy items. Pay attention to sauce descriptions—you're on the lookout for butter, cream, and oils. If you have any questions, phone the restaurant and ask for details. Once you're in the habit of doing this you will never cease to be amazed at the trigger foods restaurants sneak into the most innocuous-sounding dishes. Just because they don't list an ingredient you're trying to avoid (especially cheese) in the meal description does not mean it isn't there. Trust me, you should always ask.

Make notes right on the menu if you like, and find out if dishes can be easily altered to make them safer for you. It's usually a very simple matter for a restaurant to leave the cheese off a dish, sauté something with less oil, add extra rice or pasta or a baked potato, and put sauce on the side. When you're actually in the restaurant, order an extra basket of dinner rolls and eat several of them (choose the white bread ones, not whole wheat) to get a nice soluble fiber foundation to your meal. Remember to eat any green salads last, not first (and with a fat-free dressing), and watch out for creamy soups that start a meal (like clam chowder). Cast an especially suspicious eye on the appetizers, which for some mysterious reason are often deep fried at all kinds of restaurants. Skip those entirely unless you can find a low-fat choice hiding between the cheese sticks and onion rings.

Make it a firm habit to always ask the waiter for no dairy, no meat, and very little oil in any dish you order. I've been doing this for years and it still amazes me how much less grease there will be in my food as a result. I actually long ago reached the point where restaurant food made without a low fat request is completely unappetizing to me. You will probably find your tastes shifting along similar lines as well. I will admit that most people recoil at the thought of cheese-free pizza, but try ordering one with a lot of delicious non-meat toppings (especially roasted veggies) and give it a chance. I have unintentionally converted some friends without IBS to cheese-free pizza after they tried mine, expecting to gag, and instead loved it. On the other hand, I've also had chefs come out of kitchens because they just had to see what kind of a weirdo would order pizza without cheese. Sometimes IBS keeps life interesting in funny ways.

At ethnic restaurants, you're usually one step ahead of the game because many of them don't use dairy products at all, especially Asian places. All you need to watch out for here is fried items and hidden fat in elements like peanut or sesame sauces. Rice or rice noodles are a typical basis to Asian meals and easily allow you to follow the IBS soluble fiber guidelines. At Middle Eastern, African, and Indian restaurants pay attention to the fat content above all else. Get plenty of flatbreads for your soluble fiber and try to find grilled chicken, fish, or vegetarian choices with rice or couscous. Again, if you're unsure about an item, ask. If you're unhappy with the choices, make a special request. Be aware that French, Italian, and Greek places are typically treacherous due to their reliance on meat, cheese, other dairy, and olive oil—be extra careful here or avoid them altogether.

Remember that at restaurants you're often drinking, as well as eating, in ways you don't at home. Watch out for alcohol, carbonation, coffee, and dairy. If you're trying something new (say, a Thai iced tea, or an Italian soda) ask the waiter exactly what's in it. It's much better to be unpleasantly surprised before you order than by an attack later. For drinks, a nice trick is to take along peppermint or other herbal tea bags (see Month 2 for details) with you to restaurants. Try to order mint tea first, and if they don't have it just order hot water and brew your own. This is a really helpful tip. I promise the waiter will not hassle you about it, and you will minimize your risk of an attack.

*living*

# At Restaurants, a Friend's House, and Parties

## Restaurants—A trial run

ONCE YOU'VE scouted out local restaurants with safe and appealing choices for you, it's time for a trial run. Go by yourself or take a single close friend or family member, order an item you've previously scrutinized, take your Fibercon tablets at the table (see Month 2 to learn why), drink some peppermint or chamomile tea, then relax and enjoy your meal. You're in a no-pressure situation here, and you have prior permission to bail at any moment you feel uncertain or uncomfortable. Taking control of the situation in advance should allow you to feel at ease once you're there, and having a supportive person with you will add to your peace of mind. Once you've eaten out a few times successfully, you will gain confidence that you can *always* eat out successfully, even at a new restaurant, even with a large group. It's another example of how knowledge is power over IBS. If you know how diet can control or trigger your symptoms, you can eat as safely in restaurants as at home. You will be managing your IBS—it will not be managing you.

---

### Cheat Sheet for Restaurants

1. Order a meal based on rice, noodles, potatoes, white bread, or oatmeal.
2. *Never* assume anything on the menu is safe–ask to be sure.
3. Avoid all red meat, dairy, eggs, and fried foods.
4. Fill up on the white rolls in the bread basket.
5. Order peppermint or chamomile tea, or bring your own.
6. Divide your plate in half and eat one portion only–take the rest home.
7. Remember that drinks (soda, fruit juice, coffee, alcohol) can be triggers too.
8. Take Metamucil, Citrucel, or Fibercon before the meal (see Month 2 for details).
9. Don't be afraid to make special requests–you're the customer so you're always right.
10. Eat your green salad (with fat-free dressing) last, not first.

---

## At a friend's house

Eating at the home of a friend can be both trickier and easier than eating at a restaurant. You will be working with much more limited options, but you're also being catered to by someone who truly cares about you and has a personal interest in keeping you healthy. You will almost certainly find two sides to the coin of friends cooking for you. One, they will be very eager to prepare something safe for you that you will enjoy. Two, they will have absolutely no idea how to do so. It's up to you to give your friends the information they need to help you out, so don't feel shy about doing so.

For close friends you will be eating with often, give them this book or *Eating for IBS*. Don't feel awkward about giving them explicit information. I used to feel like I was imposing on people when they asked what special considerations they needed to make in order to cook for me. However, I gradually learned that they were sincerely interested in catering to my needs and that I was making things more difficult for them by holding back on the details of exactly what type of meal worked (or didn't) for me. Your friends and family members really want to make you a nice dinner but honestly have no idea where to begin if you don't flat-out tell them. So, tell 'em.

Tell them about your triggers and how you need to avoid meat, dairy, and fats. Let them know about the difference between insoluble and soluble fibers and what this means in practical terms of cooking a meal. Offer concrete, simple suggestions—the standard grilled fish or chicken, rice or pasta, potatoes, lots of French or sourdough breads, peppermint tea, angel food cake, sorbets. Make it clear that safe does not mean bland—it's not herbs and seasonings and flavor you need to avoid, it's the trigger foods. If your friends are interested in creative cooking, offer them IBS safe recipes that you'll both enjoy. And, to be extra careful, take your Citrucel or Metamucil (see Month 2 to learn why) right before leaving for dinner. Sometimes people have the best intentions but simply don't understand enough about IBS to offer you truly safe foods. In these situations just eat lightly of what you can, offer a gracious thank you, and plan on making your own meal as soon as you get home.

## At a party

Far and away your best strategy for eating safely at a party is to simply bring the food yourself. Odds are, the host or hostess will be happy to have you do so. As soon as you receive an invitation, call and ask if you can bring several items. Make it clear that you would like to help out but also that you have special dietary needs and it can be difficult for you to eat typical party foods. Offer a range of suggestions, from drinks to snacks to desserts, and see what appeals to your hosts. If you are planning to cook let them know what you have in mind. If the party is casual you can simply offer baked potato chips or baked corn chips, French bread, safe dips, herbal ice tea drinks, sorbets, angel food cake, fortune cookies, or homemade safe desserts. For barbecues or cookouts bring the same items and some marinated chicken or salmon steaks to throw on the grill.

In a party situation you might well simply ask yourself what you feel like eating that night, and then cater to your own appetite. You'll be happy, you'll be healthy, and pretty much all food at a party tends to get eaten anyway so you won't have to worry about whether others will like what you bring. They almost certainly will.

If you want to try the foods other people have brought, do a little detective work. Ask the host what's in a dish if you can't tell by looking. Try tiny quantities of items if you want to splurge, and make sure you've had plenty of soluble fiber first.

## FOR CHILDREN WITH IBS

*As a parent, you can easily make sure your child has safe food choices at home, but ensuring they are offered suitable foods when out of the house can be a more difficult matter. Unfortunately, the typical foods people offer children are the worst possible triggers for IBS. From burgers and fries to hotdogs and ice cream, anything that is high-fat, fried, meat, or dairy is a trigger. So are the standard children's drinks, from milk to soda pop to fruit juice. Kids often eat at their friends' houses or are taken out for fast food by their friends' parents. This is where things get sticky.*

*Children with IBS absolutely* cannot *eat at McDonald's, Burger King, or most any other fast food restaurant, because there is literally nothing safe on their menus. You need to make sure other parents know this. Your child is simply going to have to be catered to when it comes to meals and snacks, and this is a medical necessity. Hopefully other parents will be understanding and sympathetic, and willing to accommodate your children in this matter without causing them embarrassment or singling them out. This is really a pretty simple matter—lunch can be grabbed at Subway Sandwiches instead of a burger joint (make sure your child orders a chicken breast, turkey breast, or veggie choice with no cheese, mayo, or oil, and have them eat a bag of baked potato chips or pretzels with it), or a pizza place (your child can order an individual pizza with no cheese/meat) and they can have an herbal iced tea instead of soda pop. Peeled apples or bananas are good fruit options, and fortune cookies, Popsicles, or sorbets are safe desserts.*

*For parties at school teachers need to know your child requires some safe options—ask that you be notified in advance of these events so you can send baked potato chips, baked corn chips, fat-free candies (anything gummy or jelly, red licorice, jawbreakers), sorbets, soy or rice milk ice cream, herbal iced teas, and so on. You can also prepare homemade versions of junk foods—English muffin pizzas with safe toppings, Rice Krispies treats made with just a tiny bit of oil, and safe breads, cakes, pies, or puddings. Because kids can feel a lot of peer pressure to eat brown bag lunches that look like everyone else's, consider stocking up on health food stores options like safe, low-fat, veggie versions of lunch meat slices for sandwiches, soy or rice or almond cheese slices (non-dairy, not just non-lactose), soy yogurt cups, veggie chicken nuggets, veggie burgers, and so on. This way your child's lunch will look the same as it always has—the only difference will be the fact that your child can now eat it without risk of an attack.*

## IN A SENTENCE:

*In order to eat safely away from home, you'll need to plan ahead, speak up, ask questions, and make the extra effort it will take to ensure you're able to follow your dietary needs.*

*learning*

*task list*

1. TALK TO FAMILY AND FRIENDS ABOUT THE HELP YOU NEED FROM THEM TO MANAGE YOUR IBS.

2. PLAN AND THEN TAKE TRIAL RUNS OF ACTIVITIES OUT OF THE HOUSE.

3. GO FOR SHORT, THEN LONGER WALKS THROUGH YOUR NEIGHBORHOOD.

4. BEGIN TAKING BRIEF, THEN LONGER DRIVES THROUGH TOWN.

5. ATTEND AT LEAST ONE LOW-KEY SOCIAL EVENT.

# With a Little Help from Your Friends...

**IF YOU'VE** been restricting your social activities due to the fear of attacks, now is the time to carefully break out of this confinement and return to life outside your home. Far too many people end up partly or even entirely housebound when they can't control their IBS, and the sheer emotional safety this affords, despite the loss of freedom, can understandably become a habit. However, once you have your symptoms well-managed through diet and stress reduction, it's crucial that you brave the outside world and regain the active social life you were previously forced to give up. You don't have to go this route alone, fortunately. Now is the time to gather your friends and family members for a heart-to-heart talk about IBS, how you're learning to control it, and the types of help you need from them to further minimize its impact on your life.

---

### Top Ten Questions About IBS
### Your Friends and Family Need Answered

1. What is IBS? What actually goes wrong with your body during an attack? (showing them the pictures in this book might help.)
2. Is there a cure or an effective medical treatment?
3. Can you prevent IBS attacks? How can we help you do this?
4. What type of diet do you have to follow? Why?
5. Is stress a big trigger? What helps you deal with it? How can we help with this?
6. Can you still go out to restaurants? What will make this easier for you?
7. What about holidays and parties? How can we help make these occasions safe for you?
8. What would you like us to do for you when you're at home?
9. What would you like us to do for you when you're in our homes?
10. What would help you most when we go out together?

---

Are you cringing in anticipation? It's okay, I guarantee you're not the only one. Even though you know that this is a step you should take you probably feel at least a little hesitant about actually taking it. This is a real shame, and I'll tell you why. One of the worst things about IBS is not actually an aspect of the disorder itself, but the fact that the whole problem has been ignored, dismissed, and even mocked for so long. This has made sufferers reluctant (at best) to outright fearful (at worst) of telling people that they suffer from this problem. I personally kept IBS a secret from all but my closest family members and friends for over two decades. I'd make vague allusions to a "stomach problem" when I missed school or work due to attacks, and tried to deflect attention from the special food considerations I needed in restaurants or other people's homes. I felt at the time that this was absolutely necessary to save myself embarrassment or tiresome explanations in the face of blank stares and anticipated derogatory comments. However, in looking back now I wish I had been outspoken, frank, and honest from the get-go. When I look at the situation objectively, it's absolutely absurd that IBS has ever been treated as something to be ashamed of. Would I be embarrassed to have a lung disorder? Heart disease? Problems with my liver? Of course not—and I'm sure you wouldn't be either. Yet somehow, for some mysterious reason, digestive disorders as a whole are simply not accorded similar respect. With IBS, the common mistaken belief that it's a psychosomatic problem just adds insult to injury. This is wrong, and things must change. You can take heart in knowing that you are not the only person struggling with this, and you deserve to take pride in making the situation a little easier for the next sufferer by refusing to accept the status quo of being embarrassed by IBS. You've done nothing to deserve this, and you're not alone in living with it.

You will help yourself tremendously by simply telling your friends, family, and close co-workers that you have this medical problem. Give them a clear, concise explanation of the physical goings-on, let them know how severely the symptoms can affect you and restrict your entire life, and thank them in advance for their consideration and support.[4] Give them some fair expectations to live up to here and the odds are they will respond with sympathy, courtesy, and genuine efforts to help. Be open about the lack of medical treatments available for IBS and stress the importance of lifestyle factors in managing the disorder. If the people closest to you know how much you depend on the proper diet and stress management activities to remain healthy they will realize that their support can make a critical difference in your life. Let them know that this is true—don't downplay or dismiss your need for their understanding and help.

---

[4]There is a wonderful and humorous "IBS Brochure," written by a sufferer named Molly, that's available on the Internet at *www.helpforibs.com/messageboards/*. You could simply print out copies of this and give them to friends and family members as a way to break the ice with the topic.

*living*

# Become a Social Butterfly… or At Least Break Out of Your Cocoon

**THE BEST** way to ease back into social activities is slowly and carefully, with some measure of advance planning. Taking practice runs can help. The idea here is to gradually build your confidence, and realize that worries about mad dashes to the bathroom are becoming a thing of the past. You have the knowledge and the power to control your symptoms, you've taken the necessary steps to regain your health, and you now have to honestly believe that the great strides you've made will continue.

All it might take to establish the precedent of going out without an IBS incident is a single successful event. After you've accomplished that (and you will) you'll simply be building on your hard-won achievements. But wait—don't set up detailed advance plans for one important specific day, with the stress and worry that will accompany this. You don't want the social outing of a lifetime looming on the horizon—instead, start small and work stealthily.

Take a walk around your block—literally. Choose a time of day when you were previously prone to attacks, make sure you're keeping your diet and stress management routine stable, then leave the house at a time you'd normally be cautious. Take a friend or family member with you if this helps—let them know your plans and ask for moral support. Or, if having company simply sounds like additional stress, go alone at a time when your house is empty. There is no pressure on you here. No one knows you're attempting something new, and no one will know if you fail. But when you succeed, tell everyone. Get as much positive reinforcement as possible, because it's really yourself you have to convince. Physically, you've already taken the steps to control your IBS. Mentally, you still need to be persuaded by experience that your body is no longer an unpredictable enemy.

Expand your walks a little each day, aiming for a good hour in length. If it helps you to plan a route with available bathrooms along the way go ahead and do so, but tell yourself (and believe it!) that this is simply a safety precaution you will not need.

Begin to make short journeys in the car, at low-traffic hours, again allowing yourself to keep nearby bathrooms in mind so you don't have unnecessary anxiety. As your successful trips increase, vary your driving routes and times, and celebrate each outing in some little way. Every bit of progress is worth an acknowledgement and a pat on your back. Reach the point where short trips become a matter of no consequence, and are just a normal, uneventful part of each day.

Schedule a few low-key social events with a close family member or friend who's aware of your situation. Plan a trip to a movie theater or the local mall, keep the outing short and to one location, and don't build up the importance of the event in your mind. Remind yourself that there is no need for anxious anticipation or trepidation. You're simply going to go out, have a good time, and come home. Take extra precautions with your diet this day, have some soluble fiber and peppermint tea before you leave the house, and don't try to eat out. Simply go to the event and enjoy yourself.

Then plan a few longer days away from home, but choose places where you can stay in one spot for lengthy periods of time. Libraries, museums, and bookstores are good options here. They're quiet, non-stressful places with lots to do in a relatively small space, and there are bathrooms. You can spend quite a few hours here with your mind occupied by things far removed from IBS, and you won't have the anxiety of looking suspicious if you linger in any one spot. You'll be away from your house and out in public, which is a very positive step, but still in safe surroundings.

If you've joined an IBS support group (which you'll soon learn about in detail, in Month 3) and made friends, you might want to try a small group outing. You all understand each other's fears and needs, so there will be no anxiety about having to ask others to make accommodations for you. In fact, you will all likely find yourselves laughing too hard at the situation and sharing war stories to have time to worry about an attack. You'll be too busy socializing and having a good time away from home to hold onto past fears. Your goal now is to make these events so frequent that you gain the confidence to know, with utter certainty, that social outings pose no risk for you that you cannot easily overcome with a little advance planning. You're in control of your IBS at home and you can maintain this control out of the house as well. You are in the process of proving it to yourself one step at a time.

Once routine socializing becomes a normal part of your life again, make plans for more significant or challenging events. Have an evening out with dinner and a movie, confirm your attendance at an upcoming wedding or party, or take a road trip for the entire day. Realize that your success with short journeys away from home guarantees you the promise of equal success for all-day events. Just follow the same precautions with your diet, maintain your stress management program, and have confidence in the fact that you've already proven you can manage your IBS without incident away from home. Going from short trips to long ones is simply a matter of degree, not difficulty. You've long deserved to go out, be carefree, and enjoy yourself, and you now have the ability to do so. Revel in it.

## IN A SENTENCE:

> *Let your friends and family members know about your struggles with IBS, what helps you control it, and how they can support you so that you can maintain (or regain) a normal social life.*

# MILESTONE

By the end of your first month, you've now taken the steps to begin living your life normally once again on a daily basis, as you manage your symptoms while:

○ SHOPPING AND COOKING FOR THE IBS DIET

○ VENTURING OUT TO EAT AT A RESTAURANT

○ TALKING TO FRIENDS AND FAMILY ABOUT YOUR IBS NEEDS

○ BEGINNING TO RESUME A NORMAL SOCIAL LIFE

*task list*

1. **TAKE A SOLUBLE FIBER SUPPLEMENT AT LEAST ONCE A DAY, BEGINNING WITH THE SMALLEST RECOMMENDED DOSE, AND DRINK PLENTY OF WATER WITH IT.**

2. **TRY EACH HERBAL TEA IN TURN AND PICK YOUR FAVORITE, THEN DRINK IT SEVERAL TIMES EACH DAY.**

3. **CHOOSE ONE OTHER SUPPLEMENT TO TRY EACH WEEK, AND EVALUATE YOUR PROGRESS WITH EACH ONE.**

# Dietary Supplements— A Little Something Extra Can Make a Big Difference

**DIETARY SUPPLEMENTS** can be unbelievably helpful in controlling your IBS symptoms, particularly when used in conjunction with the proper diet and stress management.

Soluble fiber supplements, herbs, enzymes, calcium, and live flora cultures are the major players here, so let's take them in turn.

## Soluble fiber supplements

If you started this book on the first page and have read straight through to the second month, you've already learned how and why soluble fiber is the key to preventing abdominal spasms, diarrhea, and constipation. This is true not just for soluble fiber foods but supplements as well. So please ignore the fact that soluble fiber supplements are marketed as laxatives—they are *not*. They will of course relieve and prevent constipation, but they are just as effective at treating diarrhea, and they will not compromise normal bowel function at all once your IBS is under control. They will, however, work beautifully to keep your GI tract running smoothly, comfortably, and pain-free.

Soluble fiber supplements can be taken daily forever with no side effects or risk of addiction. In fact, they have health benefits far beyond managing IBS, as soluble fiber has been shown to lower blood cholesterol levels, reduce the risk of heart disease, and minimize colon cancer risks. Soluble fiber also slows the absorption of fats and carbohydrates into the bloodstream, which improves glycemic control and helps prevent the formation of free radicals.[1]

The most common soluble fiber supplements are Metamucil, Citrucel, and Fibercon. All are widely available at drug stores and pharmacies without a prescription. Metamucil contains psyllium, Citrucel contains methylcellulose, and Fibercon contains calcium polycarbophil. Metamucil and Citrucel are available as powders that you mix with water and drink. Fibercon is in the form of caplets. (Some people initially have bloating and gas from Metamucil and prefer Citrucel, some people can only tolerate the Fibercon pills as they can't stand swallowing the liquid supplements, others don't have a problem with any of them) From anecdotal evidence and personal experience, the powders seem to be more effective. However, the capsules are portable and more convenient, so you may want to keep a supply of both types on hand. I have Metamucil

---

[1] Dr. David L. Katz, Yale School of Medicine, New Haven, CT, presenting findings at the 1999 meeting of the American College of Nutrition, held in Washington, D.C.

in the kitchen at all times, packed into travel containers in my luggage, and Fibercon tablets in my purse, car, and office.

Try taking Metamucil or Citrucel first thing in the morning as soon as you awake, and again before dinner. Follow the dosage recommendations on the bottles and remember to start at a low dose and gradually increase your intake. Carry Fibercon tablets with you in your purse or pocket, keep some in the car, and hide a stash in your desk drawer at work. They're great to have on hand when you find yourself unexpectedly eating out, going too long between meals, or just feeling a little shaky when you're away from home. Take two capsules with a large glass of tepid water or IBS herbal tea and you'll have extra protection against attacks in dicey situations.

## Water—You Just Can't Drink Enough

**FRESH WATER** is crucial for good health in all respects, but is especially important for keeping your digestive tract functioning properly. In particular, soluble fiber requires plenty of water in order to be effective (remember, soluble fiber works by absorbing liquids in the digestive tract to form a stabilizing gel that relieves and prevents *both* diarrhea and constipation). Together, fiber and water maintain gastrointestinal muscle tone, dilute toxic wastes in the GI tract, bind irritants, bring oxygen to the tissues, and help maintain the correct balance of intestinal flora. In general, the more water you drink the better, whether plain or as IBS herbal teas. Make sure you're getting a bare minimum of sixty-four ounces (eight cups) each and every day. I routinely drink twice that much, particularly in between meals and with my soluble fiber snacks. Many Americans are actually chronically dehydrated without ever realizing it, and this is a huge exacerbating factor (and sometimes even the underlying cause) for constipation. If you're on the opposite end of the spectrum and prone to diarrhea, you're at risk of losing too much water from your body too rapidly, and this can then result in dehydration. So no matter what your IBS symptoms, and whether they're flaring or in remission, please drink up!

Make sure that your soluble fiber supplements are *not* the sugar-free variety, as artificial sweeteners can cause diarrhea in sensitive people. You may also prefer the un-dyed and un-flavored "natural" varieties, simply because it means fewer chemicals to ingest. Personally, I have no desire to put any unnecessary artificial colors and flavors into my GI tract. They may not do me any harm but they certainly aren't doing any good, so why take a chance?

Remember that different people have varying tolerances and adjustment periods to soluble fiber supplements. If you try Metamucil and feel bloated, give Citrucel a chance. If you just can't be bothered with mixing the powders at all stick to Fibercon. Do keep in mind that it can take several days to a week for your body to adjust to the increased fiber intake. Your symptoms should *not* dramatically worsen during this introductory period, and you may well see immediate improvement, but if you don't notice any difference the first day or two have patience. Soluble fiber supplements may be the single greatest aid for controlling IBS symptoms you'll ever find, so give them a fair chance.

## Herbs as medicine

The idea that herbs are nature's medicines deserves credence when it comes to IBS. There are many herbs and spices that are well-established digestive aids, most notably peppermint, chamomile, ginger, fennel, caraway, anise, oregano, and (no kidding) catnip. All are available in fresh or dried forms in grocery stores, spice shops, and health food markets. They are safe for daily use and have no risk of short- or long-term side effects.

Throughout human history the leaves, flowers, stems, berries, and roots of plants have been used to prevent, relieve, and treat illness. The history of herbal medicine is in fact inextricably intertwined with that of modern science, as many manufactured drugs used today were originally derived from plants.

The first treatise on herbal medicine was written in 2735 B.C., by the Chinese emperor Shen Nung, and this work is still in use today. The records of King Hammurabi of Babylon, circa 1800 B.C., offer instructions for using medicinal plants, including mint for digestive disorders. The entire Middle East has a rich history of herbal medicine, with surviving texts from ancient Mesopotamia, Egypt, and India that describe and illustrate the use of many medicinal plant products. Egyptian hieroglyphs show physicians of the first and second centuries A.D. using caraway and peppermint to relieve digestive upset. Throughout the Middle Ages in

Europe, home-grown herbs were the only medicines readily available, and by the seventeenth century the knowledge of herbal medicine was wide-spread. In 1649 in England, Nicholas Culpeper wrote *A Physical Directory*, and a few years later followed with *The English Physician*, an herbal manual that is still widely referred to today. The first American treatise on herbal medicine was a *Pharmacopeia* published in 1820, which included a comprehensive listing of herbs along with their properties, uses, dosages, and tests of purity. It was periodically revised and updated and in 1906 became the legal standard for medical compounds. Today's modern equivalent is the *Physician's Desk Reference*, an extensive listing of chemically manufactured drugs.[2]

The easiest and most effective way to use herbs for IBS is to brew them (fresh or dried) with boiling water into hot teas (do not actually boil the herbs in water as this can destroy their volatile oils, and thus their effectiveness). It's much less expensive to buy dried herbs in bulk and brew them with tea strainers than to purchase them as tea bags (though the effectiveness is comparable and tea bags are more conveniently portable). According to the American Botanical Council, whose mission continues the historical tradition of disseminating scientific information that promotes the safe and effective use of medicinal plants, several herbs are particularly effective for IBS: peppermint, chamomile, ginger, fennel, caraway, anise, oregano, and catnip.

For brewing teas, peppermint can be used as fresh or dried leaves; chamomile as fresh or dried flowers; ginger as a fresh root (available in the produce section of virtually all supermarkets); fennel, caraway, and anise as seeds; and oregano and catnip as fresh or dried leaves. Roughly chopping or grating the gingerroot, and crushing the fennel, caraway, and anise seeds before brewing them with hot water, will increase their strength. All of the teas can be sweetened with a little honey if you wish but they are pretty tasty plain as well. All can be chilled into iced teas also, but remember that ice-cold beverages on an empty stomach can trigger GI spasms, whereas the heat in hot teas is in and of itself a muscle relaxant.

**Peppermint:** Mint is one of the most oldest of herbs. It was used by the ancient Assyrians, and was common to the ancient Greeks and

---

[2] All information on the history of herbal medicine comes from Janet Zand's *Smart Medicine for a Healthier Child* (Avery Press, 1994).

Romans, who recognized its pain-killing properties. The mint-after-a meal custom in fact dates back to ancient Rome, and Pliny, the 1st century Roman historian and scientist, included mint in his *Natural History* in 77 A.D. Mint was not used formally in medicine until the mid-eighteenth century, but mint tea has been a favorite cure for indigestion since Biblical times. Modern peppermint is actually a hybrid of water mint and spearmint, and has stronger medicinal properties than either of the two originating plants. Internally, peppermint has an anti-spasmodic action, with a calming effect on the muscles of the stomach, intestinal tract, and uterus. As a tea, extract, or in a capsule, peppermint is useful for indigestion and GI cramps. It is anti-bacterial, increases gastric juices, and relieves gas, nausea, vomiting, and morning sickness. Peppermint also contains essential oils that stimulate the gallbladder to secrete its store of bile, which the body uses to digest fats. This makes peppermint a wonderful digestive aid for heavy meals. It also improves the function of the muscles that line the stomach and intestines, relieves diarrhea, and has a calming, numbing effect on the entire GI tract.

I find peppermint to be the strongest anti-spasmodic and pain reliever of all the herbs, and when an attack flares I really appreciate its noticeable whole-body mild anesthetic effect as well. On a daily basis I find it more effective (and certainly more enjoyable) than prescription anti-spasmodic drugs, particularly when it's brewed very strong. In fact, peppermint is such a powerful muscle relaxant that it can trigger GERD (Gastroesophageal Reflux Disease) or heartburn in people who are susceptible. *If you are prone to these upper GI problems, avoid mint in all forms and stick to the other herbs and spices.*

Peppermint is also available in other forms that can be truly beneficial to IBS. Enteric-coated peppermint oil capsules are available in some health food stores under varying brand names, and can be ordered through the mail as well.[3] Taken before meals they help prevent symptoms and have no side effects. Even Altoids, the "curiously strong" peppermint candies, can have a soothing effect on the gut. I've been known to pop them before or after meals as a safety precaution, either chewing them or just swallowing a couple whole. Fresh breath and no IBS—what more could anyone want?

---

[3] Peppermint Plus brand enteric-coated peppermint oil capsules can be ordered from *www.totaldiscountvitamins.com*, or 1-800-283-2833. Pepogest brand capsules are available at *www.iherb.com*, or 1-888-792-0028, and at many U.S. health food stores.

To make peppermint tea, simply brew 1–2 tablespoons dried (or 3–4 tablespoons fresh) mint leaves per eight-ounce cup of fresh boiling water.

**Chamomile:** The use of chamomile dates back twenty-five hundred years to ancient Egypt. In 500 B.C., Hippocrates, the founder of modern medicine in ancient Greece, recognized the therapeutic properties of chamomile. Ancient Egyptians, Romans, and Greeks used chamomile flowers to relieve colic. The herb is an official drug (recognized by government authority) in twenty-six countries. Chamomile has anti-spasmodic, anti-inflammatory, anti-peptic, anti-bacterial, anti-fungal, and sedative properties. It has been used for centuries in teas, and extensive scientific research over the past twenty years has confirmed many of the traditional uses for the plant, and established pharmacological mechanisms for its activities. Used internally, chamomile is known for its calming effect on smooth muscle tissue, making it an effective remedy for gastrointestinal spasms and menstrual cramps, as well as GI tension resulting from stress. Chamomile is also used for indigestion and gas. It's often taken as a bedtime beverage, due to its mild sedative effects. *Chamomile is a member of the daisy family, which means that anyone who is allergic to other members of the daisy family, including ragweed, should not use it. If you are unsure about this, please consult your doctor or allergist.*

Brew 1–2 tablespoons dried (or 3–4 tablespoons fresh) chamomile flowers per eight-ounce cup of fresh boiling water.

**Ginger:** The use of ginger dates back to ancient India, China, and Japan, where it's been cultivated for thousands of years. Ginger was sold to the ancient Greeks and Romans by Arabian traders, the Spaniards brought it to America, and it's now grown in the West Indies. Chinese herbalists have been recommending ginger for more than twenty-five hundred years, and it plays an important role in traditional healing in cultures around the world. Ginger is helpful for a wide variety of gastrointestinal ailments ranging from simple indigestion to severe nausea and cramps. It provides effective relief for morning sickness and post chemotherapy nausea, and has been shown to be more effective for preventing motion sickness than Dramamine. If you've overeaten at a meal, ginger is particularly helpful, as it contains very powerful digestive enzymes. It can also increase your appetite before a meal. Ginger acts as an anti-spasmodic, helps prevent vomiting, and improves the tone of intestinal muscles. It also has a mild anti-inflammatory action. When ginger is applied topically to the skin it increases blood flow to the area and acts as a mild pain reliever.

Brew 1 tablespoon (about a 1" chunk) fresh crushed gingerroot per eight-ounce cup of fresh boiling water. Gingerroot itself can be boiled without losing effectiveness.

**Fennel:** Fennel's use is documented in ancient China, and the plant is mentioned in virtually every European work on herbal medicines from ancient times to the present day. The mild licorice-flavored herb is native to the Mediterranean, was known to the ancient Greeks, and was spread throughout Europe by Imperial Rome. In the first century A.D. Pliny attributed twenty-two healing properties to fennel. According to Chaucer, the fourteenth-century English poet, fennel was one of the nine holy herbs of the Anglo-Saxons. The herb has anti-spasmodic properties and it stimulates the production of gastric juices. It's useful for bloating, gastro-intestinal and menstrual cramps, gas, diarrhea, colic, heartburn, indigestion, and stomachaches. The U.S. once listed fennel as an official drug to be used for digestive problems, and today the herb is still used daily as an after-dinner digestive aid from India to Italy to Spain.

Brew 1–2 teaspoons fennel seeds per eight-ounce cup of fresh boiling water.

**Caraway:** The use of caraway seems to date to the ancient Arabs. The ancient Greek physician Dioscorides noted that the seeds aid digestion, and throughout history in Europe, the Middle East, and early America, caraway was a favorite addition to laxative herbs because it tempered their often violent effects. It was also used for menstrual cramps. Medicinally, caraway has been used to treat indigestion, nervous disorders, and colic. To this day, in countries around the world, caraway is a traditional ingredient in foods such as meats and cheeses that are heavy and difficult to digest. Caraway has an anti-spasmodic effect as well as anti-microbial properties, and it stimulates the production of gastric juices. Two chemicals present in caraway seeds (carvol and carvene) soothe the smooth muscle tissues of the digestive tract and help expel gas.

Brew 1–2 teaspoons caraway seeds per eight-ounce cup of fresh boiling water.

**Anise:** Anise is an ancient spice indigenous to the Mediterranean. It was cultivated by the Egyptians, Greeks, and Romans, and noted in the works of Dioscorides and Pliny. Anise has been grown in Italy continually since Roman times for use as a digestive aid. Anise was introduced to central Europe in the Middle Ages and by the fourteenth century was so popular in medieval England that King Edward I placed a special tax on the spice to raise money to repair London Bridge. The seeds have a very sweet, pronounced licorice taste and contain a volatile oil, *anethol*, that aids in the digestion of rich foods and settles the stomach. Anise stimulates gastric juice production, relieves nausea, and is helpful for colic. It regulates digestion, making it useful for both constipation and diarrhea. Anise is helpful for belching, gas, bloating, vomiting, chronic diarrhea, gastrointestinal cramps, and sluggish digestion. It's also a mild sedative and is useful for calming stress-related nervousness and relieving insomnia. The spice has anti-spasmodic and anti-fungal properties, and helps prevent fermentation and gas in the stomach and bowels.

Brew 1–2 teaspoons anise seeds per eight-ounce cup of fresh boiling water.

**Oregano:** The use of oregano is documented by the ancient Egyptians, the Greeks used it for convulsions and muscle cramps, and the herb is mentioned by Aristotle as an antidote to poisoning. Traditional Chinese medicine has used oregano for centuries to relieve vomiting and diarrhea. Early American colonists brewed the leaves for muscles cramps and stomach troubles. Oregano contains two volatile oils, *thymol* and *curvacol*, that act as anti-spasmodics, increase the production of gastric juices, ease bloating and gas, and relieve menstrual cramps. Oregano aids nausea and morning sickness, and has a calming effect as a muscle relaxant. The dried or fresh leaves of the herb make a warm, spicy tea that will probably remind you of pizza. Oregano oil has anti-spasmodic, anti-convulsant, pain-killing, anti-inflammatory, and antiseptic properties. Pure oregano oil can be found at health food stores and through internet sources[4] and is typically taken by adding 2–4 drops to a cup of hot water or herbal tea. Enteric coated capsules are also available. The pure oil should never be used undiluted

Brew 1 tablespoon dried (or 3 tablespoons fresh) oregano per eight-ounce cup of fresh boiling water.

---

[4]The Web sites *www.sheld.com* and *www.greatamericanproducts.com* both carry pure oregano oil.

**Catnip:** Catnip, a perennial mint, was initially cultivated by the ancient Greeks and Romans, who used it for insomnia. From the Mediterranean it spread north across Europe and by the Middle Ages was widely grown for a seasoning and as a drink. Catnip arrived in America with the early colonists and was a garden staple, used to brew tea for upset stomachs and to aid sleep. The herb calms the digestive system, and is particularly safe and useful for children. Catnip has anti-oxidant and anti-inflammatory properties, and is a powerful anti-spasmodic that helps relax the entire intestinal tract. It relieves gas, heartburn, and colic. It's also believed to assist the nervous system by way of its influence on the digestive system, and is a mild sedative and mood-enhancer. The herb is also effective for tension, anxiety, and insomnia, again particularly in children.

Brew 1–2 tablespoons dried (or 3–4 tablespoons fresh) catnip leaves per eight-ounce cup of fresh boiling water.

Since discovering herbs for IBS just a few years ago (I sure wish I'd known about them sooner), I've become positively addicted to peppermint tea. Now I buy the herb from my local health food stores for about six bucks a pound, and this quantity lasts me a good two or three months. I drink several cups a day, every day, and I carry peppermint tea bags with me whenever I travel. I do like to brew chamomile and anise every once in a while for a change of pace, and sometimes to accompany specific ethnic foods (anise sweetened with a little honey is wonderful with Indian and Middle Eastern meals, and it's also delicious with chocolate). Overall, I've found herbal teas to be one of the easiest, fastest, safest, and downright enjoyable remedies for preventing and halting the entire spectrum of IBS symptoms, and I would urge you to give at least one of them a try.

## Avoid at All Costs

**AS AN** aside here, the worst possible herb for IBS is tobacco, which is a GI tract stimulant, irritant, and carcinogen. Talk about three strikes and you're out. Please don't smoke it or chew it, and try to avoid rooms filled with it. Your colon will thank you.

## *Other pills to pop*

Soluble fiber and strong, hot herbal teas are usually very effective supplements for controlling IBS. There are a few other options to explore in this area as well, and they're very safe and healthy overall so you definitely don't have much to lose by trying them.

**Digestive enzymes** may be helpful when taken right before a meal, especially if there is more fat in that meal than is safe for IBS. Enzymes are available at all health food stores and may be of more benefit to older people, as natural digestive enzyme production declines with age. A related product, Shaklee Peppermint-Ginger Plus, is a digestive aid with a combination of peppermint, ginger, fennel, and anise that has received some enthusiastic support from IBS sufferers.

For gassy foods such as beans, lentils, and many vegetables, there is Beano, a brand-name digestive enzyme. Beano contains the sugar-digesting enzyme that the body needs (and which some people lack) to digest the complex sugar *raffinose*. If you have trouble digesting raffinose the sugar will ferment in your colon, producing gas and intestinal distress. Beano breaks down raffinose into simple sugars that cause no GI discomfort. Beano is available as tablets or drops, and is simply taken at the beginning of a meal.

**Acidophilus supplements**, which are live cultures, are available as pills or in soy yogurt (avoid dairy yogurt). These cultures help normalize and maintain healthy gastrointestinal flora, which can minimize diarrhea. They are most effective when your gut is under assault from antibiotics. Acidophilus supplements (make sure the label says "live cultures") are widely available at drug and health food stores, and should be stored in the refrigerator. Take the supplements with food.

**Calcium** plays a critical role in regulating muscle contractions, and it also has a constipating effect. As a result, calcium supplements (1500 milligrams a day) can be truly beneficial for people with diarrhea-predominant IBS. In particular, Caltrate and Caltrate Plus have had spectacular results for some folks, and have a lot of anecdotal support for their use. Remember that calcium can block iron absorption in the body and contribute to anemia, so women who take calcium supplements may want to take an iron supplement at a different time of day. Calcium should be taken with food. Do *not* take antacids containing calcium—all antacids have a laxative effect.

**IN A SENTENCE:**

> *Supplements such as soluble fiber, herbal teas, digestive enzymes, live flora cultures, and calcium can be of tremendous benefit to controlling IBS.*

# MONTH **3**

*task list*

1. JOIN OR START AN IBS SUPPORT GROUP.

2. SET ASIDE SPECIFIC TIMES TO PLAN AND
   EVALUATE YOUR ONGOING STRATEGIES
   FOR DEALING WITH IBS, AND TRY NOT TO
   DWELL ON THE PROBLEM OUTSIDE THESE
   TIMES.

3. MAKE A HABIT OF TREATING YOURSELF TO
   THINGS THAT MAKE YOU HAPPY.

# Support Yourself— You Are NOT Alone

**IT'S YOUR** third month after diagnosis, and you're probably just now coming to terms with the fact that you have an
incurable illness. Hopefully you've spent the past two months
gradually adopting the various lifestyle strategies that will
allow you to control your IBS, and your condition is rapidly
stabilizing, but you may still be dealing with symptoms that
range from uncomfortable to unbearable. The weight of taking
responsibility for managing the disorder on a daily basis, for
possibly the rest of your life, falls solely on your shoulders. You
likely need a break.

This is a good time to remember that there are millions of people out there struggling to overcome IBS just as you are. They're facing the exact same problems, asking the same questions, and trying the same strategies. You do not have to go through this alone—you can meet them. Burdens are always easier to bear when you can share your worries, compare experiences, and just find some comfy shoulders to lean on. Talking about IBS, how to deal with it, and exchanging innovative means to overcome it is a great way to give yourself the support and comfort you need when you're newly diagnosed. Joining an IBS support group is one of the easiest ways to get this kind of help.

There are quite a few support groups already in existence in America and Canada, and more are forming every day. There is a terrific internet resource, The IBS Self Help Group, founded by IBS sufferer Jeffrey Roberts, that has a live chat session every Wednesday and Sunday evening at 8:30 P.M. EST. You can become a member for free at Yahoo and join the group at *http://clubs.yahoo.com/clubs/ibsselfhelpgroup*.

> *"I intend to establish IBS Self Help Groups across the United States, Canada, and the United Kingdom, so that individuals who are suffering from this disorder can get face-to-face support from each other."*
>
> —JEFFREY ROBERTS, Toronto, Canada, President and Founder of the IBS Self Help Group, age 40, IBS sufferer since age 7.

*"As a child I had constant stomachaches, constipation, and diarrhea, and was taken to the doctor numerous times. I was given mineral oil and suppositories, and dairy was almost eliminated from my diet, in an attempt to regulate my bowel movements. I was also labeled as 'sensitive' and as having a 'nervous stomach' due to my complaints.*

*In grade school I had a great deal of difficulty in the mornings due to cramps and diarrhea. During school tests I would hurry to finish so that I could run to the bathroom. I didn't know a different way of living, but I did know that I didn't feel well.*

*At the age of fifteen I was diagnosed with lactose intolerance. Removing dairy completely from my diet instantly took away some of the nausea and diarrhea that I suffered. However, diarrhea, cramps, and constipation did continue. The cramps became more intense and interfered with my lifestyle. I began to associate what I ate and drank with how I felt. Wherever I went I carried anti-spasmodic and anti-diarrheal medications. I still had not been diagnosed with IBS, but I began to go from doctor to doctor in search of a diagnosis and cure.*

*By age seventeen, I had constant diarrhea with alternating consti-pation, and a feeling of butterflies in my stomach. I was prone to a sudden, recurring, knife-like pain in my lower left side that would cause me to double over in agony. After meals I felt very bloated and my gut was really noisy. I felt ill first thing every morning, but could improve as the day progressed. I was nervous about socializing due to fear that I would have a sudden urge to go to the bathroom or would be struck by the knife in my gut. This was a lot for a teenager to deal with, let alone try to cope with on top of all the other challenges of growing up. For years now my family doctor had ruled out a number of illnesses via basic tests, and although he was always willing to lis-ten to me, he was still unable to solve the problem or make a confi-dent diagnosis. He now referred me to several gastroenterologists. The first GI doctor suggested that since I was a 'sensitive' person, my pain and illness were all in my head. He performed a very painful sigmoi-doscopy in his office, in a very rude and uncaring manner. No positive results came from this exam.*

*The second gastroenterologist was at a larger hospital, and he too seemed annoyed by my lack of more 'serious' symptoms but he suggest-ed a number of tests. He performed an even more painful sigmoi-doscopy, then joked that because of my thin appearance he should send me to McDonald's for fattening up.*

*I had now turned eighteen years old, and the third GI doctor I saw listened to me and seemed truly interested in how I was feeling. He did some blood work and performed a gastroscopy followed by another lac-tose intolerance test. He was confident that I did not fit the diagnosis for any gastroenterological disease. He diagnosed me with IBS, and he wanted to treat my symptoms with diet and medication. He prescribed Tagamet, then the miracle drug for ulcers. I soon went off to universi-ty at age nineteen and felt very unwell over this entire year.*

*After several severe flare-ups over the course of the next several years in university, my GI doctor suggested a colonoscopy. Given my past expe-riences with the brutal sigmoidoscopies, I was too nervous to submit to* this exam. Instead I changed medications every three months trying to find the magic combination.

By age twenty-two I had stopped pursuing medical help, but was eventually forced to seek another opinion due to recurring IBS flares of pain, diarrhea, and constipation. One day as a young adult, while at my first professional job as a computer software developer, I developed the familiar intense knife-like pain. I walked into the emergency room of a nearby hospital. Here I found a new doctor who performed my first of three colonoscopies, as well as another gastroscopy and barium enema. This doctor's attitude was that if I didn't obey her dietary rules then she wasn't interested in having me as a patient. This was not the type of doctor/patient relationship I was looking for. Nonetheless, her diagnosis once again confirmed IBS.

I still could not believe that anyone could live with so much pain, diarrhea, and constipation without having a more definable illness, so I sought opinions from two other specialists. They both confirmed the diagnosis of IBS. During this time I continued to do my own research, and tried to take charge of my symptoms. At the age of twenty-five I was finally becoming comfortable with the IBS diagnosis. Over the next several years, during times of crisis, I continued to see the doctor with whom I had the best relationship.

During this time, from my own experimentation and research, I learned how to use fiber to fill my gut and try to control the pain, diarrhea, and constipation. I also came to terms with the fact that IBS is a chronic illness with no cure. I learned to 'roll with the punches' and tried not to anticipate the worst or overreact to the onset of symptoms. I discovered that pain in my gut was a signal that I should go to the bathroom, and I learned which foods might trigger a bout of pain, diarrhea, and/or constipation.

When I started to take charge of my illness I read everything I could find about IBS—unfortunately, there wasn't much to be found on the subject. In 1987, at age twenty-six, I began attending monthly meetings of a newly formed IBS Meeting in Toronto. I became more involved in the group and eventually led it, as I felt motivated to help others as well as myself. The meetings died out as attendance dwindled, but I reworked the group into a phone support line and published occasional newsletters, continuing in this vein for seven years. In the *meantime, at age thirty-two, my own IBS continued to wax and wane. After yet another severe flare-up I had one more colonoscopy, which again confirmed the IBS diagnosis. I began to take a low dose anti-depressant that at first made me so tired my teeth were numb, but which eventually helped control my pain and diarrhea. I stayed on this drug for a year, and was relatively symptom-free.*

*In 1994, I created a small Web site (as a computer professional I had the access and skills to be my own webmaster), which described Irritable Bowel Syndrome. I listed the few books and drugs available for the illness. Within a year I had two hundred members in my IBS internet group. In May of 1995, I created a new Web site and the IBS Self Help Group, as it's known today, was born.*

*As the Web site grew, I found that people were very concerned about the loneliness the illness imposed, as well as the symptoms of diarrhea and constipation. Many people were confused about what they should or should not eat, and I was constantly asked for diet information. I heard from so many people who found reassurance in just knowing that there were other people out there who felt the same way they did. Many simply wanted validation that IBS is a real illness. Some of the people I heard from were completely housebound and were hoping to gain confidence that they could overcome the illness. As a result of numerous conversations with fellow sufferers, I started an IBS bulletin board on the Web site so that individuals could share their concerns and knowledge with others. My work as administrator of the IBS Self Help Group was now becoming a second career.*

*The Web site continued to grow and eventually gained the attention of pharmaceutical companies and medical researchers. I kicked off a self-help group in New Jersey and gave advice to new support groups in Los Angeles, New York, and Vancouver, B.C. I began to attend IBS medical conferences and quickly learned all of the latest research. My role as administrator grew to President, IBS Self Help Group.*

*However, my own IBS continued to flare. I lost weight and became very ill. The workload of my two full-time jobs was now taking its toll on my health. At thirty-nine, I had yet another colonoscopy with a new GI doctor, which yet again confirmed the diagnosis of IBS. I adjusted my diet to try and control my symptoms, and once more was prescribed antidepressant and anti-spasmodic medications to manage the pain* and diarrhea. I filled these prescriptions but never actually took the drugs, because from past experience I knew the side effect of fatigue would not allow me to work at the pace I needed.

At this same time, the pharmaceutical company GlaxoWellcome introduced the IBS drug Lotronex to much fanfare. The IBS Self Help Group was featured on their patient brochure and in the drug labeling, and the Web site experienced sudden explosive growth. When Lotronex was pulled from the market I helped members of the IBS Self Help Group create the Lotronex Action Group, which seeks immediate re-access to the medication. Concurrently, the pharmaceutical company Novartis was having difficulty obtaining FDA approval for their IBS drug Zelnorm, and many IBS Self Help Group members sought my help in getting access to that medication. In response, I launched the Zelnorm Action Group, which seeks the immediate release of the drug.

Recently, in order to fill the gap between IBS researchers, doctors, and patients, I've established the Irritable Bowel Syndrome Association. This is a nonprofit organization dedicated to helping everyone who suffers from IBS through patient support groups, treatment, accurate information and education. I intend to establish IBS Self Help Groups across the United States, Canada, and the United Kingdom, so that individuals who are suffering from this disorder can have face-to-face contact with each other.

Today, at age forty, my own IBS continues to be troublesome and to interfere with my work, lifestyle, and family. I no longer fear socializing as most people know about my chronic illness, and I use medication for the pain or diarrhea only when absolutely necessary, but I do still occasionally become overwhelmed by the illness and depression when I suffer a severe flare-up. At least now I better understand how my body works. Recently, I attended a presentation at a gastrointestinal conference for IBS. I thought to myself that although I was there to take notes and ask questions for the IBS Self Help Group, I was also really there for myself. I do want to live a 'normal' life. I want to get better and I am incredibly motivated to do whatever it takes to get there.

In the meantime, it is of no small consolation to me that I am able to help others with the IBS Self Help Group. The Web site continues to provide extensive, accurate, and current information, and I am *proud to say that it has grown to become the premier organization for IBS sufferers. It currently has in excess of seven thousand registered members from across the world, and the Web site receives over 2.2 million visitor hits per month. I'm sent roughly fifty e-mail messages per week from new IBS sufferers around the globe looking for answers to their problems. I try to tell them all that I know what they're going through, and that although there may not be a cure yet it is encouraging that research is being performed which might one day determine the cause of IBS. With a cause, a true cure (or at least a method to cope) is sure to be found."*

If you would like to meet with others in person, check the side bar for a support group in your area. If you don't see a local option, check the Support Groups page at *www.helpforibs.com/supportgroups/* for new listings, or call your local hospitals and ask if they have any groups in existence.

If you can't find a nearby support group, start your own. What, just like that? Yes! If you have IBS, you have the sole qualification required to begin a new support group. Even if you decide to invite guest speakers from medical, dietary, or stress management fields, it's crucial that a patient (like you!) lead the group, as only someone with IBS knows exactly what it's like to live with the problem. You may want to restrict the group to other IBS sufferers or open it to family members and close friends who are looking to help loved ones. Your group can have multiple objectives, from sharing symptoms and remedies to discussing the latest medical research.

All you—the newest IBS support group leader—need really do is set a time, find a location, and do some minimal advertising. You can ask your local hospital, community center, library, or public school if they have space you can use. Once you have a set location, call your family doctor and gastroenterologist and let them know about the new support group. Contact local hospitals and GI clinics and inform them as well, so they can pass the information onto patients. Print up some simple flyers on your (or a friend's) home computer, and send them to the hospitals and clinics, post them at libraries and community centers, and ask your local paper to run a public notice. You don't need to use a graphic designer or print shop for this project, simply keep things nice and neat (and well-proofread), and

# IBS Support Groups

## America

### California (San Francisco) IBS Self-Help Group
When: The first Thursday of each month
Time: 6:00 P.M.–7:00 P.M.
Place: St. Mary's Medical Center, 450 Stanyan St., San Francisco, CA
Cost: $10
Contact: Womankind at 415-750-5775

### California (Southern California) IBS Support Group
When: The first Saturday of each month
Time: 11:15 A.M.–1:00 P.M.
Place: St. John's Hospital in Santa Monica, CA
http://home.switchboard.com/ibs
Contact: Frank Brown, fbrown627@yahoo.com

### New Jersey IBS Self Help Group
When: The first Friday of each month
Time: 7 P.M.–8 P.M.
Place: Overlook Hospital
99 Beauvoir Ave. (off of Morris Ave.), Conference Room #1, Summit, NJ
Contact: New Jersey Self Help Clearing House 1-800-367-6274

### New York (Middletown) IBS Connection
When: The fourth Tuesday of each month
Time: 7:30 P.M.
Place: Horton Medical Center
60 Prospect Ave., Conference Room #C, Middletown, NY
Contact: 1-800-HORTONMD

### Oregon (Portland) IBS Support Group
When: January 10, 2001
Time: 7:00 P.M.–8:30 P.M.
Place: West Hills GI, 9155 SW Barnes Rd. Suite 635, Portland, OR
www.westhillsgiresearch.com
Contact: Jerri Pawson/Liz Welch, research1@westhillsgi.com

# IBS Support Groups

## Canada

### British Columbia (Kelowna) IBS Support Group
When: The last Tuesday of each month
Time: 4:00 P.M.
Place: Kelowna General Hospital, Lecture Room—Rose Avenue entrance
Contact: Marian 250-762-8984

### British Columbia (Port Moody) IBS Support Group
When: The first Tuesday of each month
Time: 7:30 P.M.
Place: Eagle Ridge Hospital, Lower Level across from cafeteria
475 Guildford Way
Contact: Marilyn 604-942-6059

### Toronto IBS Self Help Group
When: The last Thursday of each month
Time: 7 P.M.–8 P.M.
Location: Mount Sinai Hospital, 600 University Avenue, (University Ave
south of College Street), Room: 15th floor classroom
Contact: Jeffrey Roberts, ibs@ibsgroup.org, 416-932-3311

use brightly colored paper or a similar eye-catching feature. Remember that the more professional your flyer appears, the greater the likelihood that people will respond to it.

If you have a community help-by-telephone assistance program for human services (such as 2-1-1), call and ask them for self-help clearing-houses serving your area (they may be able to assist in advertising), and also ask to have your new support group added to the database of referrals for other callers. A great internet resource for starting a support group can be found at *http://mentalhelp.net/selfhelp/startup/newgroup.htm*. Once you've got your group established, you can also publicize it at the largest IBS site online by e-mailing Jeffrey Roberts at ibs@ibsgroup.org with your information. He'll list your site on the IBS Self Help Group's web page, *www.helpforibs.com/messageboards/*.

When it's time for your first meeting, keep things short and sweet. People can simply introduce themselves, give a brief personal history, and share their objectives. The goal is mutual support, so keep everything casual and comfortable and let people get to know each other. Establish the time for your next meeting, gather e-mail or phone numbers for everyone, then call it a night and go home flush with success. Congratulations—you've just established your very own IBS support group, and it will be tremendously helpful for you as well as everyone else who joins it. Good job!

Do keep in mind that all groups will experience slow times when there is low attendance, but don't get discouraged. Simply keep in touch with your members, take a short hiatus if necessary, and re-advertise to expand the group. Whether you're the leader or simply a member, any support group experience is sure to be helpful, reassuring, and rewarding.

In addition to support from fellow IBS sufferers, you need to support yourself when you're newly diagnosed with IBS. It's important that you treat your health as a priority, and devote the time and energy needed to take care of yourself while you learn about IBS and begin to manage your symptoms. So give yourself a break—lots of them. Set aside a time to plan your strategies for dealing with IBS—you can follow the day/week/month format of this book—and outside that time try not to dwell on the problem. Give yourself permission to stop worrying, take one day at a time, and say no to people and projects for which you simply don't have the time, energy, or interest. Treat yourself in small ways, every day. You need comfort as well as support—so no guilty feelings allowed. Do make sure you let your family and friends know that you've been diagnosed, give them an overview of IBS so they understand what you're going through, and don't be afraid to ask for their help and sympathy (hopefully you've already had success in this area after following Week 4). Now is not the time to stoically shoulder your problems alone. Go ahead and lean on the people closest to you while you learn how to control your symptoms—you'll be glad you did.

## FOR CHILDREN WITH IBS

*I sympathize so much with children who have IBS. I've had it myself since the fourth grade, so I know exactly what they're going through—and it's not fun. It is much easier to deal with the problem as an adult, for quite a few reasons. Primarily, most people have the habit of not taking children seriously, whether regarding what they claim they can or cannot eat, or discounting the very real stress they often endure. Kids are labeled as fussy or difficult much more readily than adults, and they are often not shown the common courtesy that they deserve. People can treat children with a lack of respect they wouldn't dream of showing other adults. As a result I have quite a few vivid memories of horrific IBS attacks that could have been prevented entirely had adults simply bothered to listen to me, so I would urge parents to insist that their children be given the special consideration IBS can require. This is a legitimate, physiological disorder, and it needs to be taken seriously. IBS is not somehow a more minor problem just because the sufferer happens to be a child. Kids with IBS need support even more than adults, and it's really up to their parents to make sure they get it. They will likely face many situations where they will not be able (or allowed) to adequately speak for themselves, so it's up to you to speak for them. Their health depends on it.*

*Parents have to help their children deal with IBS in two areas: their life at and away from home. At home you have the unimpeded ability to make life safe for your child by preventing exposure to IBS triggers. Away from home you must protect them as well, and this is more difficult. It's quite likely that the single most important thing* you can do to help your children manage IBS is to stand up for them against other adults. Children don't have the power to stand up for themselves—adults just don't give them the credibility they give other adults.

There may well be times when your child simply cannot physically tolerate a stressful situation. If this happens it might be easier to just eliminate the trigger than struggle through ongoing attacks. Children with IBS can sometimes need permission to quit. If they're taking a class at school and, for whatever reason, find it intolerable, let them drop the class for another option if at all possible, or at least switch to a different teacher. If there's a specific teacher they want to avoid up front, make a special request so they're placed in a class environment that's comfortable for them. If public speaking is a huge stress trigger and they're forced to give oral presentations, let their teacher know how difficult this project is for them, and assure your children that you'll understand if they don't do as well in this area.

Reassure your children that their health comes first, and that while you obviously want to see them excel in all aspects of their lives, you also realize that there may be times when, despite their best efforts and good intentions, IBS might compromise them. You may actually be surprised in this regard by how much of a difference it can make in your children's stress levels if they know you'll understand a failure that results from IBS flares beyond their control. Ironically, with some of the stress removed from these situations by your lowered expectations, they're actually much more likely to do well. This is also the type of situation they're almost certain to outgrow, so have some patience and be tolerant—they are, after all, still children.

There may also be times when children need to bow out of a situation completely. If they are stuck in a class, on a sports team, or in an after-school activity that is causing them great stress and making them literally sick, get them out of that situation immediately. As a parent you have the power to step in and do this, and if it's what your child needs (and wants), please do it for them. These occasions are likely to be rare, and you do need to have a heart-to-heart talk with your child to ensure they never cry wolf in *this matter, but when their need is legitimate don't hesitate to rescue them. They're likely not able to rescue themselves.*

*My parents' support in this manner was invaluable to me when I was in school. They had a hands-off policy in general, but if I asked them to step in for me, they never hesitated. Knowing they were always there when I needed them (but wouldn't ever interfere without my knowledge) gave me tremendous reassurance and peace of mind. In return, I tried never to ask for their help unless I had no alternative and was unable to fight my own battles any longer.*

*In 8th grade in particular, there was an extremely stressful situation that became completely intolerable to me and had drastic effects on my health. My fourth period class was band, and it was taught by a teacher who terrified me. He often screamed at the entire class for up to an hour straight, randomly singled out students to play solos which he would then brutally criticize, and forced all the students to play through lunch (which immediately followed his class). Students routinely left his room in tears. I began to dread band to such an extent that I was having attacks almost every single day during 3rd period due to the stress of anticipation. Several times each week I had to go home from school mid-day, doubled over in pain, because of how that class affected me. My parents became increasingly alarmed but I asked them to let me try to handle the situation on my own.*

*However, things eventually reached the point where I was simply unable to bring myself to endure that class one more day. As I struggled through yet another horrible hour in 3rd period, watching in dread and increasing pain as the clock ticked off the minutes, something inside me finally snapped. Fourth period arrived, I marched to the front office, and announced to the school counselors that I was never going to set foot in band class again. A huge uproar ensued because it was against school policy to drop a class mid-semester (though apparently not against policy to terrorize twelve-year-olds and forbid them to eat lunch).*

*To my everlasting gratitude, my parents immediately stepped in at my request, as I was now clearly in over my head. They were forced to spend an entire week in meetings with the band teacher (who was astonished to learn how he was affecting me), school counselors, and the utterly terrifying Principal Tupton. They were told I might be expelled if I did not return to band, to which they replied that attending a class that made me physically ill was not an acceptable option. At the final meeting, my grandmother (I was raised by my grandparents) actually stood up, told the principal he was not listening to her, and walked out of his office. My grandfather followed. To this day I cannot mentally picture that scene, as my grandmother was the most polite, elegant, kind, and considerate woman I've ever met, and the principal was a seven-foot ogre famous for two things: physically intimidating students, and never, ever smiling. (I still occasionally run into people from junior high who remember me simply as the girl whose grandmother stood up to Tupton.) At the end of the week, the school relented and I was permitted to drop the class. My daily IBS attacks immediately ceased. Do I still play a musical instrument? No. Do I regret this? A little. Do I regret dropping band? Not for one minute. After all, it can be difficult to blow a saxophone when you're vomiting from pain.*

*Having the support of my parents in this situation actually gave me the courage to continue standing up for myself, and to speak out when I was under stress beyond the limits of what I could physically endure. Knowing that I always had the option to walk away from overwhelming situations gave me the freedom to pursue interests that involved risks (for me, public performance activities like drama and running for class office). I knew that no matter what the outcome, I would always come home to a hug from my grandmother and her reassurances that as long as I had tried my best, she was proud of me. Thanks to her unwavering support, though I wasn't always able to overcome stressful circumstances, I did became quite confident at facing them and usually things went very well. Having a back door open and the knowledge that I could leave at any time was a key to success for me. Many times I simply wouldn't have tried something new at all had I not had an escape route. The risk of neverending IBS attacks would have been too great a threat to ignore, and one that was definitely not worth taking.*

*Even with the support of wonderfully sympathetic and supportive parents, however, I often went through hell dealing with IBS as a kid. Other adults frequently insisted that I eat foods I knew made me terribly ill, or casually dismissed concerns causing me severe stress-related attacks as "not worth worrying about," simply because they thought I was just whining. They did not believe I had a medical problem even when I flat out told them so. Please try to shield your children from similar experiences. Let them know that you will defend and fight for their health at every turn. Children with IBS who cannot rely on the sympathy, understanding, and unwavering support of their parents stand a much greater chance of losing the battle before it begins.*

## IN A SENTENCE:

*Look to support from fellow IBS sufferers, and support yourself as well when you're newly diagnosed with IBS, because you must devote the time and energy needed to take care of yourself while you learn about IBS and how to manage your symptoms.*

# MONTH **4**

## task list

1. VISIT YOUR DOCTOR FOR A FOLLOW-UP
   APPOINTMENT.

2. POINT OUT ANY NEW SYMPTOMS OR
   CONCERNS THAT MAKE AN IBS DIAGNOSIS
   QUESTIONABLE.

3. REQUEST NEW PRESCRIPTIONS IF YOUR
   CURRENT MEDICATION IS NOT WORKING TO
   YOUR SATISFACTION.

4. IF YOU'RE NOT HAPPY WITH THE MEDICAL
   CARE YOU'RE RECEIVING FOR IBS, MAKE
   AN APPOINTMENT WITH A NEW DOCTOR.

# Follow Up with Your Doctor

BY NOW you should have your diet and stress levels well under control. Hopefully, you have also found a prescription medication that is helpful for at least some of your symptoms, some of the time. However, you may have quite a few new questions about IBS now that you've had some time to live with it and try to successfully manage your symptoms. This is the time to make a follow-up appointment with your GI doctor and get those questions answered.

If you weren't happy with the gastroenterologist you saw previously who actually diagnosed your IBS, by all means see a different one this time around. Let your new doctor know when you received your diagnosis and how you've been dealing with it. Talk about what prescription medications you've already tried, if you've found one that works better than others, how tolerable you find the side effects, and what medical help you feel you still need to manage your symptoms. Ask if there have been any new developments in IBS research, clinical findings, or drug advancements that may help you. You can view your doctors as partners, not autocratic authorities, in managing your treatment plan, and you can fairly expect them to see your relationship in a similar light.

If you have joined or started a successful support group, found a particular diet or stress management strategy highly effective, or developed an innovative way to control your symptoms, let your doctor know. What has worked for you is quite likely to work for others, and your doctor probably has many other patients still struggling with IBS. Helpful hints that you share may well benefit other people facing your same problems.

If your symptoms have changed or new symptoms have developed since your diagnosis, stress these points with your doctor and make sure that your IBS diagnosis is truly valid. You may warrant additional tests at this point. Remember that, while IBS itself cannot develop into more serious diseases, it is possible that you may find yourself facing a new and entirely separate health problem that needs to be addressed. In particular, if you have noticed blood in your stool, upper GI distress, fever, or joint swelling, you should insist on a new round of diagnostic tests. Additionally, for anyone who self-diagnosed themselves with IBS, I'd urge them once again to have their suspicions confirmed by a board-certified gastroenterologist. No matter how unnecessary this seems it is a crucial step to take, as it's worth gaining the peace of mind of that will come from knowing there is truly nothing more "seriously" wrong with your health than IBS.

If you are faithfully following the IBS diet, a stress management program, taking supplements, and trying prescription medications but still have not had a dramatic improvement in your symptoms, it's time for a second (or third, or fourth) medical opinion. IBS is well-managed through these lifestyle modifications. If you are not significantly better at this point you may not have IBS after all. It's time to find out.

## IN A SENTENCE:

> *If you have any new questions or concerns about your IBS, or have developed new symptoms, make a follow-up appointment with your GI doctor.*

*task list*

1. **PLAN A HOLIDAY CELEBRATION WITH TRADITIONAL FOODS ADAPTED TO BE SAFE.**

2. **MAKE THE MEAL YOURSELF, BRING SAFE FOODS TO THE PARTY, OR ASK THE HOST AHEAD OF TIME TO MODIFY RECIPES PER YOUR SUGGESTIONS.**

# Time for a Holiday— Let's Celebrate!

**GETTING YOUR** IBS under control on a day-to-day basis is simply a matter of learning the ground rules and assimilating them into your normal routine. Keeping yourself stabilized then becomes a part of your daily habits, which are probably fairly consistent. But who wants to live a life with each day monotonously like the one before, without any special occasions and celebrations?

By now you're ready to move on to managing your IBS symptoms outside the daily grind, and tackle a holiday celebration. Do you have a sinking feeling in the pit of your stomach at the very thought? Don't worry, that's understandable. It's quite likely that, from experience, you tend to anticipate holidays with dread instead of excitement simply because you've found yourself suffering attacks in the midst of the festivities many times before. This is pretty common, and was certainly the case for me for many years. Easter brunch...bolt to the bathroom in the middle of the egg hunt. Christmas dinner...agonizing cramps before the presents were even all opened. Hardly the stuff of which fond memories are made, as you surely know all too well.

However, looking back now it's clear that most holidays posed many obvious dangers. Unfortunately, I was totally oblivious to them at the time. Normal eating habits go right out the window when you're celebrating—party foods are usually richer than your average meal, and portions are often much larger (more Thanksgiving turkey with extra gravy, anyone? And have a third slice of that pecan pie while you're at it). Add to the dietary triggers the stress of traveling to your destination or hosting the festivities yourself, dealing with possibly strained family relationships, the disruption to your comfy daily routine that holidays bring, the poor night's sleep that's likely to follow, and the anxiety born of past mid-celebration attacks. It's no wonder that so many special occasions result in IBS flare-ups. The good news? You can prevent IBS symptoms as effectively during a holiday as you can for any run-of-the-mill day of the week. The better news? You don't have to miss all the great food or any of the fun to do so.

As with all other special events in your life, you'll have to plan ahead and take precautions to prevent IBS symptoms. This requires a bit of time and effort, true, but the payoff is well worthwhile. For any holiday that revolves around food (and, honestly, don't they all?) the more say you have in the dishes prepared, the more safe choices you'll get to eat. This may mean having the party at your house, and doing the cooking yourself. If this is a possibility for you, give it serious consideration. Total control is a lovely thing when it comes to eating for IBS.

For the food itself, simply modify your traditional family favorites following the IBS dietary guidelines you learned in Week 2. If some of the must-have dishes are inherently triggers (Christmas roast beef, say, or Fourth of July fried chicken) go ahead and prepare them as is for your guests, but add in some tasty substitutions for yourself (start a new tradition of a boiled Yule lobster, and barbecue skinless chicken breasts for that summertime picnic). You'll likely find that many of your holiday standbys can be altered with minimal effort and delicious results—honest. For years now I've been making my own IBS version of my grandmother's traditional Easter brunch with a scrambled egg and veggie dish (now with egg whites and soy cheese), lemon sticky bread (low-fat, high soluble fiber), salmon spread on bagels (the cream cheese base is a tofu variety, not dairy), and fresh fruit salad (which I eat last). Do I tell my family that they're no longer eating precise versions of my grandmother's recipes? Are you kidding? I operate on a strict need-to-know basis when I cook for guests. As long as they think the food's delicious, that's all they need to know.

## IN A SENTENCE:

> *You can prevent IBS flare-ups during holiday celebrations without giving up great food and fun, by just controlling your diet as you do every day and modifying traditional family recipes according to the IBS dietary guidelines.*

# Holiday Foods—Safe *and* Scrumptious!

**COOKING A** big family holiday meal can be overwhelming even when you're not keeping IBS dietary triggers in mind. Luckily, there are many fast and easy ways to safely substitute or modify most traditional holiday foods without spending an extra moment in the kitchen, such as:

## EASTER

BRUNCH: French toast made with soy milk/egg whites, browned with cooking oil spray in a nonstick skillet, topped with maple or fruit syrups. Scrambled egg whites or tofu with sautéed wild mushrooms or mild salsa. Low fat chicken, turkey, or salmon sausages. Bagel selection. Fresh fruit smoothies (no dairy) instead of whole fruit salad. Hot peppermint tea instead of coffee.

DINNER: Roast chicken or Cornish game hens instead of lamb. Roasted new potatoes and steamed spring vegetables. Lots of fresh crusty French bread. Banana creme pie with graham cracker crust, substituting soy milk for dairy and egg whites for whole eggs in the custard.

## PASSOVER

Matzo balls made with egg whites only and veggie broth, added to low fat chicken soup. Potato kugel (try sweet potatoes) made without oil, using just egg whites. Low fat sponge cake made with matzo cake meal and potato starch, topped with stewed strawberry rhubarb compote.

## FOURTH OF JULY AND SUMMER PICNICS

Barbecue skinless chicken breasts, catfish or salmon fillets, soy hotdogs, or Gardenburgers. Baked potato chips and baked corn chips. Potato salad made with fat-free mayonnaise (spike with fresh lemon juice and herbs) and hardboiled eggs without the yolks. Herbal ice teas instead of soda pop. Angel food cake instead of biscuits for strawberry shortcake. Soy/rice milk ice cream or sorbets.

## THANKSGIVING

Roast a turkey but only eat skinless white meat, no gravy. Mashed potatoes without butter or whipping cream (use soy milk), with a few roasted garlic cloves blended in. Stuffing made with veggie broth instead of oil, no sausage. Candied sweet potatoes with very little oil, or baked squash topped with brown sugar. Pumpkin pie with graham cracker crust, use soy milk instead of dairy, substitute 2 egg whites for each whole egg.

## HANUKKAH

Potato latkes browned with cooking oil spray in nonstick skillet. Top with lox and fresh dill or homemade cinnamon applesauce. Surround a dark chocolate cake (substitute applesauce for most of the oil, use a recipe with cocoa powder instead of solid chocolate, replace each whole egg with 2 egg whites, and use extra vanilla extract to heighten sweetness and richness) with gelt and top with edible gold foil.

## CHRISTMAS

For appetizers, make favorite dips for fat-free crackers with soy sour cream or tofu cream cheese to replace dairy, and try low fat hummus or fruit salsas. Cold boiled prawns with cocktail instead of tartar sauce. Baked whole salmon or boiled lobster instead of a roast or goose. Low-fat rice pilaf and roasted root vegetables. Chocolate angel food cake (made with cocoa powder—you can just add $\frac{1}{4}$ cup to a packaged mix) with fruit sorbet or a seedless raspberry sauce. Make a variety of low fat fruit breads (banana, zucchini, pumpkin) to mix in with the Christmas cookies.

If someone else has kitchen duty for your next holiday, ask the cook in advance what dishes you can prepare and bring with you. Go ahead and bring a few other things that you like and can safely eat as well—no one will complain that there's too much food at a holiday celebration. You may also have surprisingly good luck with simply asking your family cook to modify the recipes for you, or cook a few special dishes that meet your dietary needs. You probably know well in advance what the traditional meals are for your family celebrations, so spend some time considering what steps can be taken to make these dishes safe for you, then share your suggestions with the host. It doesn't take any special cooking skills or practice to substitute soy milk for dairy in that special holiday brunch French toast, or to make Thanksgiving stuffing minus the sausage and with veggie broth for moisture instead of butter. A few sleights-of-hand along these lines in the kitchen and you will be able to eat with confidence. Now, there's a true cause for celebration!

# MONTH **6**

*task list*

1. MAINTAIN ALL SUCCESSFUL STRESS
   MANAGEMENT STRATEGIES.

2. DISCONTINUE ANY UNHELPFUL THERAPIES,
   BUT TRY TO DETERMINE WHY THEY FAILED.

3. IF YOU HAVEN'T YET FOUND A GOOD FORM
   OF STRESS MANAGEMENT, RE-EVALUATE
   ALL YOUR OPTIONS AND CHOOSE
   SOMETHING APPEALING, THEN BEGIN
   PRACTICING IT IMMEDIATELY.

4. MAKE AN APPOINTMENT FOR THE FIRST
   SESSION OF AN ALTERNATIVE THERAPY
   YOU HAVEN'T YET TRIED.

# Re-Evaluate Your Stress Management Strategies and Alternative Therapies

**NOW IS** a good time to take a step back and re-assess your stress level, as well as your ability to cope with it. You have hopefully established the habit of practicing some form of daily stress management. How is it working for you? Did you choose a method that is maintaining its appeal as well as its effectiveness? Just what is its level of effectiveness, anyway?

Set aside a block of quiet time to really consider how your stress-related IBS attacks compare today to what they were two months ago. You should be seeing significant improvements by now, and have gained the confidence of knowing that you can expect to see increasing benefits as your practice continues. If you have achieved these results, develop a plan to ensure things continue along this path. If you've been taking classes that have been helpful, make it a priority to have the time and money to participate well into the future. Ask yourself if there are any routes to further improvement, and what steps you need to take to achieve this. Try to anticipate any problems that might arise, and plan now for how you could solve them.

If you like the method you chose and feel hopeful that it could help you manage stress, but have found obstacles in the way of regular practice, take the time to determine why. Make two lists—what you need to reach your practice goals, and everything blocking this achievement. Then make a concerted effort to determine how to either solve the problems you've listed or work around them. Remember that this is your health at stake, and you are truly deserving of whatever commitments are required to get results. Time, money, and resources may need to be spent—and you're worth it.

If your new stress management technique is just not working for you, or if you've already abandoned it completely, re-assess your needs and interests in this area. Figure out exactly what you didn't like and why you were unable to maintain your practice—and be honest with yourself. These reasons are only for you, no one else has to approve, so don't worry about how "legitimate" your complaints may seem. I hate fluorescent lights and can't bring myself to work out in a gym that has them. Silly? Probably. But it's enough to keep me from exercising, and therefore a valid reason to make sure I only join gyms with good lighting. This might mean one that costs a little more, or is a few minutes farther from home, but if the result is that I'll actually make the effort to get there, well, that's what truly matters. The end justifies the means in this case.

If you determine that something specific was problematic for you in maintaining your new stress management practice, accept this and focus on figuring out how to work around it. If you just didn't like the activity you chose, and feel this is an inherent problem not related to a poor teacher or scheduling difficulties, choose another type of practice and decide what you need to get started. If you tried yoga and hated it, be honest with yourself about why and choose a new option that's very different. Maybe traditional exercise is a more appealing option to you—weight lifting? racquetball? swimming? Pick one and give it a shot. If you sort of liked your activity but didn't totally love it, try something else along the same lines but just a little different. Perhaps switching from a traditional Tai Chi class to a kung fu session that includes Tai Chi practice will spark your enthusiasm.

If you think you may have found a good activity but just ran into too many problems to practice it, make a list of the reasons why. Then take an honest assessment of what you can do to solve these problems and give your chosen activity another chance. If time constraints are a problem, try switching to a class or gym closer to home. If just finding the energy to throw on workout clothes and leave the house is tough, rearrange your living room furniture so there's enough space to workout in front of the television and buy some appealing videotapes. Don't like to miss your favorite programs by watching a tape? Get a treadmill and put it in front of the television so it's staring you in the face. If money is a concern, consider lower-cost alternatives, such as segueing from a yoga class to following a yoga tape. Whatever it takes is whatever you need to do. Remember that stress management is a priority, and you should seriously try to find the time and resources to practice some activity every single day. After all, your IBS isn't going anywhere, so your stress reduction definitely should be.

Have you tried acupuncture or hypnotherapy? Are you happy with the results? These treatments can take a few months to result in significant improvements, but you should certainly know by now if the therapy is working. If you're not impressed with the outcome, consider trying an alternative.

You may wish to simply see a new practitioner, or you might want to switch approaches altogether. There are acupuncturists in every town these days, and some health insurance plans even cover them. If you haven't gone this route yet, look around for someone who has experience with IBS patients and understands the disorder, and give them a chance to help you. Ask them for patient references so that you can talk to someone with IBS who has already had the treatments and experienced successful results. You may want to choose an acupuncturist who offers Chinese herbal medicine as well.

If you have not yet tried hypnotherapy, consider giving it a go. If you're interested but know that you honestly will just never get around to finding a qualified therapist in your area, let alone make it to a series of appointments away from home, take another look at the *IBS Audio Program.* Without having to make much effort at all here you can try a treatment that's racked up truly impressive success rates. It doesn't take much to order the tapes and you can listen to them in the comfort and privacy of your own home. This is one of the only forms of alternative therapy that you don't have to find time to leave the house for. The tapes are shipped to your door, and you listen to the program at whatever time of day is quiet and convenient for you. If you know this is probably the only way you'll ever realistically make the time and effort to try an alternative therapy, give it some serious consideration. There's little to lose and much to gain.

If you're intrigued by an alternative therapy I haven't addressed, feel free to go ahead and give it a try. From biofeedback to aromatherapy to therapeutic massage, holistic approaches are gaining in both popularity and mainstream acceptance. And truthfully, most of them are quite enjoyable ways to spend some free time. There is rarely any risk of side effects from these types of treatments, and there is always a very real chance of success, so pursue your own interests in this area. The fact that most alternative therapies have no track record when it comes to treating IBS is more likely a function of the fact that so little research has been conducted in these areas, not a prediction of their failure. If you feel hopeful that a new approach to your IBS management program might help you, don't hesitate to try it. If you're interested in exploring other avenues but aren't sure where to start, if you have Internet access *yahoo.com's* alternative health section, for one, is chock-full of great information and resources for finding professionals in your area. You could also check *about.com* under the Alternative Health and Alternative Medicine categories. You might also simply call your health insurance company and ask what alternative therapies, if any, they cover (in some states such coverage is legally required).

If you have no reluctance about giving alternative therapies a chance, but haven't yet done so, odds are the reason is that you just haven't gotten around to it. These therapies often fall into the category of "sounds like a good idea, wish I had the time to check it out." If you're guiltily recognizing yourself right about now, don't feel too bad. We all, even after decades of dealing with IBS, likely never exhaust every possible avenue of treatment. Researching an alternative therapy, finding a practitioner, setting aside the money, and simply finding the time for routine appointments can delay the best intentions.

If this is the case, schedule time on your calendar—right now—for investigating the alternative therapy of your choice and choosing a practitioner. Remind yourself that your health is a top priority, so dedicate the funds and time to follow through on this matter. Consider the therapy appointments a private treat, and view them as something to look forward to for the pleasure of the experience itself (most alternative therapies are at a minimum very relaxing, and might well be downright heavenly). Anything that gives you a break from daily hassles and your too-busy world is quite likely to make you feel healthier and happier in general, and have at the least an indirect impact on your IBS symptoms. If the treatments have a direct effect as well, that's better still. Either way there's nothing to lose by trying—except your IBS. I'll bet you won't miss it.

**IN A SENTENCE:**

> *Evaluate your stress levels and related IBS attacks, and if you haven't seen improvements re-assess your current program, take a new approach, and consider trying an alternative therapy if you haven't already.*

# MILESTONE

*Now that you're halfway through your first year with IBS, you've regained your health and resumed a normal social life, and have:*

○ FOUND THE MOST HELPFUL SUPPLE-
MENTS FOR YOUR SYMPTOMS.

○ JOINED OR STARTED AN IBS SUPPORT
GROUP.

○ FOUND A PRESCRIPTION MEDICATION
THAT HELPS YOU.

○ CELEBRATED AN IBS-SAFE HOLIDAY.

○ ARRIVED AT A SUCCESSFUL STRESS
MANAGEMENT STRATEGY.

*As you now enter the last half of the year, you can expect to relegate IBS concerns to the background of your life, and:*

○  **BECOME COMFORTABLE SPEAKING UP ABOUT IBS AS A HEALTH ISSUE.**

○  **TAKE A VACATION.**

○  **RE-EVALUATE YOUR SUPPORT SYSTEM.**

○  **KEEP CURRENT WITH IBS RESEARCH.**

○  **EXPLORE ETHNIC, VEGETARIAN, AND HEALTHY CUISINES.**

○  **REVIEW THE PAST YEAR AND YOUR ACCOMPLISHMENTS.**

*task list*

> 1. CONTACT YOUR LOCAL MEDIA AND ASK THEM TO COVER IBS IN THEIR HEALTH NEWS.
>
> 2. LET YOUR HUMAN RESOURCES DEPARTMENT AT WORK KNOW ABOUT IBS AND HOW MANY EMPLOYEES IT'S LIKELY AFFECTING, AND ASK THEM TO DISSEMINATE INFORMATION ABOUT THE DISORDER ALONG WITH TIPS FOR MANAGING SYMPTOMS.
>
> 3. JOIN AN INTERNET MEDIA CAMPAIGN OR IBS SURVEY GROUP.

# Make Your Voice Heard— Why You Should Talk About IBS

ONE OF the most frustrating things about living with IBS is the persistent feeling that you alone have this problem and no one else really understands it. Hopefully you joined a support group in Month 3 and no longer feel like the only person in the world with your symptoms, but you are probably still running into plenty of people who have never even heard of IBS, and who think you're either some kind of medical freak or that the problem is all in your head. I'm not sure which of these attitudes is worse, but I do know that it gets plenty tiring dealing with either one of them. IBS is one of the single most prevalent health disorders around. You are *not* alone. The condition itself, as well as the basic lifestyle modifications needed to manage it, should be common knowledge akin to knowing the rudimentary facts about diabetes or asthma. After all, IBS affects more than twice as many people than these other health problems *combined*.[1] So why do you still have to deal with the frustration of feeling all alone with a disorder you must constantly explain to people as if it were some exotic tropical disease? Maybe it's time to take a stand on this issue and have your voice heard.

Taking some concrete action to "get the word out" about IBS, its impact on people, and how it has directly affected your life can be tremendously empowering. Don't be afraid to stand up and be counted, to let people know that IBS is a serious, legitimate medical problem, and that you would like to see some attention paid to this issue.

Consider writing to your local congressperson and asking him or her to lobby for additional funding for IBS medical research. Contact your local print, radio, and television media, and request that they cover this topic and bring the issue into the public eye. If you work for a large company visit the human resources department and let them know there's a tremendous need for employee/employer education on the topic (give them the "IBS is the second leading cause of worker absenteeism" statistic and watch their eyes widen in surprise). There are online campaigns at IBS Web sites (*www.eatingforibs.com*) attempting to bring national media coverage to the issue—why not add your voice to the chorus? If you haven't already, join an Internet IBS support board to rant, find friends, or just get a sympathetic ear when you need one.

---

[1] 17 million people in the US have asthma [National Institute of Health Centers for Disease Control and Prevention. CDC Surveillance Summaries. *Morbidity and Mortality Weekly Report* 47, SS–1 (April 24, 1998)]. Seven million to fifteen million people in the U.S. have diabetes [National Center for Health Statistics. *Vital and Health Statistics Series* 10, no. 200 (1996)]. It's estimated that up to fifty million people have IBS (IFFGD—*www.iffgd.org*).

You can also participate in the ongoing Internet DrugVoice IBS survey and join the IBSVoice Panel (*www.drugvoice.com/ibs.htm*). This survey gives you an unparalleled (and totally anonymous) chance to vent about your experiences with IBS, provide feedback on prescription and over-the-counter drugs, and discuss other treatment options. I participate in the panel on a regular basis and find it both interesting and very cathartic. DrugVoice is a for-profit consumer research and marketing company specializing in taking the patient's perspective, as voluntarily supplied by panels of active health care consumers (like you), to pharmaceutical and health care leaders. The information they gather is used to develop health care products, treatments, and clinical trial protocols. DrugVoice partners with a variety of organizations to access patients interested in participating in the DrugVoice panels. In exchange, DrugVoice provides these organizations with access to research findings. You will likely find it quite empowering to sound-off about IBS while knowing that you will be listened to by major pharmaceutical companies, physicians who treat IBS patients and conduct research, and even the FDA.

In the end, I hope you'll realize and take to heart that IBS is not something to be ashamed of, embarrassed by, or hidden. For too long people with this problem have suffered in silence, and this has only perpetuated the lack of respect, attention, research, and treatments for the condition—much to the detriment of those of us dealing with it. Take direct action to change this situation, to stand up for yourself personally, and to draw attention to IBS in a larger context. You are part of an enormous group of people—millions of them—enduring the same vicious symptoms and resultant lifestyle restrictions. IBS is not your secret, it should not be relegated to the shadows and spoken of only in whispers, so share the problem with the world and a solution for all of us is much more likely to follow. This is truly one way in which helping yourself is guaranteed to help others. And that is always a good thing.

**IN A SENTENCE:**

> *It can be empowering to make your voice heard, so speak up about IBS and explore avenues to bring it into the public eye as a serious, physical disorder that millions of people, including you, live with.*

*learning from living*

*task list*

1. PLAN A VACATION, AND FOR A NEW
   DESTINATION RESEARCH WHAT TO EXPECT
   IN TERMS OF LOCAL CUISINE, EATING
   TIMES, SLEEPING HABITS, AND CLIMATE;
   ASSESS WHETHER OR NOT YOUR IBS
   NEEDS CAN BE ADAPTED TO THESE
   SURROUNDINGS.

2. CHOOSE A SOCIAL ENVIRONMENT THAT
   WILL MAKE IT EASY FOR YOU TO MAINTAIN
   CONTROL OVER YOUR SYMPTOMS.

3. STOCK YOUR LUGGAGE WITH
   SOLUBLE FIBER SUPPLEMENTS, SAFE
   NON-PERISHABLE SNACKS, AND HERBAL
   TEA BAGS.

4. DETERMINE IN ADVANCE HOW YOU CAN FIT
   YOUR STRESS MANAGEMENT PROGRAM
   INTO A VACATION ROUTINE.

5. TAKE THAT TRIP AND ENJOY YOURSELF.

# Take a Vacation

NOW THAT you have your day-to-day life well under control, you've earned the confidence to try a break in your routine—in other words, it's time to plan a vacation. Whether you take a weekend road-trip to the nearest beach or a month-long bike ride through Holland, you'll need to put a little thought into your itinerary and take a few extra precautions to manage your IBS when traveling.

The best part of most vacations is joining in activities, from food to music to sightseeing, that aren't common where you live. However, a sense of routine can be crucial to maintaining control over IBS symptoms, so you'll need to strike a happy balance between new experiences and stability. All of the normal stress factors of vacations—the travel itself, irregular meal times, disrupted sleep, sharp climate changes, and so on—can trigger attacks under the best of circumstances, so in terms of IBS, vacations are actually a time to give more, not less, thought to controlling your symptoms.

You may want to explicitly choose a type of vacation that will enable you to manage your IBS in the easiest ways for you, and in the surroundings you find most comfortable. This might mean taking a cruise, so you have very little travel to-and-fro as well as your own private room to retreat to at any time. You'll also have a tremendous variety of food choices, built-in accessibility to exercise facilities, and a convenient, quiet bedroom for mid-day naps to ensure you stay well-rested. You can travel with a group of close friends and have happy, stress-free socializing built right into your trip. Plus, there are lots of bathrooms nearby for peace of mind. On the other hand, hiking out into the wilderness and pitching a tent under the stars might offer the most relaxing holiday you can imagine. You can bring all of your own food, have absolute privacy, no activities to plan or crowds to deal with, and day hikes will pleasantly provide all the exercise you need. You also have the great outdoors around you at all times so proximity to bathrooms is not a concern.

Suit yourself here, from peace and quiet in nearby mountains to arts and culture in a foreign city. Travel alone, with just a loved one, or a wide circle of family and friends—whatever you find most comfortable. Don't even try to plan a vacation with elements that you know up front will leave you frazzled. Make a safe stable diet, stress management, and good sleeping habits your priorities and build a suitable holiday around these factors. A wonderful vacation (with no need for bathroom proximity after all) is sure to follow.

In terms of diet, your destination will likely dictate what you'll be able to eat, and the degree of difficulty you'll face. Take this into account in advance and, even if you don't expect trouble, pack emergency rations of soluble fiber foods (dry cereals and packets of instant oatmeal work beautifully) and supplements, as well as plenty of peppermint tea bags. Read travel books and talk to friends to learn exactly what you can expect for overseas destinations. What are the country's food staples? What are their common meals and snacks? What are their meal times? Do these fit into the IBS diet or not? If they don't, what are your alternatives? Are there ethnic restaurants you can opt for? Markets where you can shop instead of relying on restaurants? Safe street food? What are the kitchen facilities, if any, in your hotel room?

Don't be afraid to choose safety over authenticity. You may be one of the few tourists in Dublin searching out Japanese restaurants, but at least you'll stay healthy. In almost every vacation destination there are bound to be some traditional foods that perfectly fit your needs, from baguettes in France to fresh tortillas in Mexico to rice in Hong Kong. Go ahead and splurge on local specialties that are safe IBS staples—then stock your hotel room, carry a small stash with you during the day, and treat yourself to frequent snacking opportunities.

I know it can be hard to resist going native and downing Turkish coffee when you're in Istanbul, or plates of schnitzel in Austria (and temptations are especially strong when everyone else is indulging), but remember that even though you are on vacation your IBS is not. You, unfortunately, cannot leave your cranky colon behind while you traipse around the world. Just remember that this does *not* mean you therefore don't get to traipse around the world, or that you can go but you won't be able to enjoy it.

As usual with IBS, it just means taking some time to think things through in advance. It will be well worth your while to make careful but flexible plans, take some simple precautions, and prepare to ask questions or make special requests on your trip to get your dietary and stress management needs met. By the way, feeling guilty about somehow being "difficult" in this regard is not allowed. Taking care of your health is a legitimate priority and that's that.

For the travel itself, whether car, plane or train rides, bring your own food—lots of it. Do not assume that the meals being provided by travel services, or the tourist restaurants along your route, will offer any safe choices whatsoever. Odds are they won't. It's very important that you are extra careful to follow the IBS dietary guidelines from the first day of your trip to the last, as travel is virtually always upsetting to your body even if you're not immediately aware of the effects. This physical stress can quickly rear its ugly head in the form of an IBS attack if you allow it, so concentrate on prevention at all costs.

The power of precautionary measures is what will enable you to enjoy your vacation, not suffer through it.

> *"My whole trip was great and I had a wonderful time,*
> *thanks to following the IBS diet guidelines."*
>
> —DIANE FEIERABEND, age 64, Lake Elsinore, California,
> IBS sufferer for over 30 years.

*"I first started having problems with IBS long before it was even iden-tified as such. I had a serious bout with a flu bug around 1968 and spent a week in bed, then almost three weeks recuperating. I thought the ongoing diarrhea I had was a result of the flu and paid no atten-tion, until it continued for several years. At this point a doctor described my problem as primarily due to stress, which seemed reason-able given that I had four active kids, had started working full time, had lots of bills to pay, and there were problems in my marriage. A friend of mine was also having serious problems with diarrhea and her doctor prescribed Metamucil, which she swore by. I found a new GI specialist and asked about using Metamucil but he told me that was a 'stupid thing to do' because it was for constipation, not diarrhea, and that I should stop using it. After a full GI workup I was once again told my problem was all due to stress and I just needed to relax. Yeah, right! My life basically had to be planned around avoiding social events like dinner and theater, dinner and a movie, or dinner and **anything**, and I was always looking for the location of bathrooms. Needless to say, traveling was extremely difficult.*

*Only in 1999 when I had access to the internet was I finally able to get some rational information about IBS, as well as learn the name for it. Getting the* Eating for IBS *diet information was the most beneficial element. For the first time things made some sense, I became aware of the difference between soluble and insoluble fibers, and what a differ-ence that makes! I was finally able to travel again, and my daughter and I went to Hawaii in October 1999. I followed the IBS diet guide-*

*lines and packed my own snacks and lots of water for the plane trip. I took dry cereal, fat-free crackers, hard candy, and bottles of water. I passed on the airline food (do they really call it food?) altogether. In Hawaii I was delighted to find that plain cooked white rice is available everywhere, even at McDonald's of all places, so I ordered white rice with almost every meal we ate. I avoided the salad bars and for breakfast I made oatmeal from packets I had brought with me. We had a full kitchen in our hotel so this was easy. I just used a coffee pot to heat water and made oatmeal that way. Even at a luau on Maui there were lots of things I could eat, using rice as my staple. If I filled up on rice first then I would not be so tempted to overeat other foods. The entire trip was great and I had a wonderful time, thanks to the IBS diet guidelines. Whenever I travel now, either by plane or auto, I always take a snack pack with dry cereal and fat-free soda crackers, plus lots of water. I continue to use Metamucil, mostly once a day. I will up it to twice daily when traveling, so if I'm bingeing off the diet it helps at those times. Just recently I took a cruise to the Mexican Riviera and made a real effort to stick with the diet. No salads, careful fresh fruit choices, I ordered a baked potato almost every dinner, and mostly ate the fish entrées instead of meat. I did indulge in the desserts, even a couple of chocolate pig-outs. On the cruise rice was also offered at the buffet on deck for every meal so this was my first choice before anything else. I didn't even need the Metamucil the entire cruise and I had very few problems. When I follow the diet I am just fine."*

In addition to taking dietary precautions, maintain your stress management program while traveling, or at least a modified version of it, to the best of your ability. You may have to replace morning aerobics with evening walks, find a quiet corner of your campsite to regularly practice meditation or yoga, or ensure in advance that your hotel and room are in a quiet location so your sleep is uncompromised. Do whatever it takes, and feel free to substitute any alternative that works for you. Exercise is one of my daily methods of stress management, and I insist on time for it while on vacation, but I'm flexible about how this is managed. Though I jog regularly at night at home I find this totally impractical while on a holiday (although I know others who manage to fit in a daily run wherever they go). Instead, I typically spend each day sightseeing via long walks everywhere, and I invariably log many more miles on vacation than I do on my evening runs. The end result is the same—great exercise and resultant stress reduction and relaxation—so it doesn't matter if the method differs.

If exercise is key to your IBS management as well, make it a priority to stay in lodging with a gym, pool, weight room, or whatever else you require. Take your work out clothes and shoes with you and unpack them first so they're staring you in the face. If you don't have the option of exercising as planned once you're actually on your vacation, change tactics and adapt—find any variation that works and run with it. Maintenance is the key here and flexibility will get you everywhere.

Disruptions to your sleep cycle are common when traveling, particularly if you change time zones. Make an extra effort to overcome this potential trigger as quickly as possible. If you fly overseas you may want to write off the first day entirely and just sleep through it. Yes, you'll lose some valuable vacation time up-front, but this initial loss will be more than offset by the stability you'll gain for the rest of your trip. If you can, pack your own pillow whenever you travel, and you'll likely sleep much better. Check the bed in your hotel room as soon as you arrive and if it's not satisfactory, speak up. If the bed is truly dreadful consider changing hotels. As a daily rule, try to go to sleep earlier than you think necessary and get a little extra rest—this will definitely minimize your risk of attacks. Even scheduling a few naps here and there can make a world of difference. Vacations are supposed to leave you well-rested, after all.

Remember that travel is one of the single most stressful tests for people with IBS, and as a result even the best laid plans to prevent attacks can go awry. Try hard to keep your sense of humor in the face of this. The likely worst-case scenario is that your precautions will fail to result in total success and you'll experience minor symptoms. But if disaster strikes and you become far more intimately familiar with, say, the Vatican bathroom than the Sistine Chapel ceiling, ride it out, then pull yourself together, dust yourself off, and remember that an attack is the exception, not the rule. You know how to break the cycle through rest and diet, so give yourself the next day off to regain stability. One bad incident won't ruin your entire vacation if you refuse to let it.

I once became desperately ill on a long train ride in Wales and spent the entire journey (through lovely, castle-dotted countryside—or so I was told) doubled over and vomiting from pain in a tiny, incessantly rocking bathroom. I eventually missed my stop and had to get off the train and double back. Did this ruin my trip? Do I now despise the Welsh? No, of course not. I reminded myself that few things are truly disastrous in the broad scheme of things, and had faith that if I simply soldiered on and took steps to stabilize myself, I could continue my vacation without further incidents—and that's exactly what happened. It's still not a happy memory, but one I tried hard to find some humor in and conquer in my own way by relegating it to where it belonged—as a single, isolated incident in an otherwise fabulous and healthy vacation. For three weeks spent traveling through four different countries without an itinerary, my IBS remained stable every day except that one. Overall, I had a wonderful time, saw beautiful sights, and immersed myself in delicious cuisine from dim sum in London's Chinatown to grilled salt cod along the coast of Portugal. I came home just a little tired but already eagerly anticipating my next vacation. No, the trip wasn't perfect, but it was delightful, and I refused to be afraid to take another one. Don't you be either.

Bon voyage!

## IN A SENTENCE:

> *A routine is crucial to managing IBS, and the inherent stress factors of travel require giving careful thought and planning to how you'll maintain control over your symptoms while on vacation, but the rewards are well worth the extra effort.*

*task list*

1. FORGIVE YOURSELF IF YOUR VIGILANCE SLIPS AND YOU TRIGGER AN ATTACK.

2. DON'T BE TOO DISCOURAGED IF YOUR IBS FLARES DESPITE YOUR BEST EFFORTS— JUST REMIND YOURSELF OF ALL THE SUCCESSFUL STRATEGIES YOU'VE FOUND FOR CONTROLLING YOUR SYMPTOMS, REMEMBER THAT THERE IS ALWAYS ANOTHER OPTION TO TRY, AND THEN SIMPLY REGROUP AND CONTINUE TO GO FORWARD.

3. TALK TO FRIENDS AND FAMILY WHO AREN'T QUITE GIVING YOU THE SUPPORT YOU NEED, AND LET THEM KNOW YOU REALLY DO NEED THEIR HELP.

# Take Stock of Your Support System... Especially When You Fall Off the Wagon

**WE'VE ALL** done it before. We'll probably all do it again. The lifestyle restrictions that IBS imposes can at times seem too tiresome and just not worth the bother…so we simply stop following them. This is particularly likely to happen when things are really going well, because it's human nature to tell yourself that since everything's fine right now it will surely just continue that way. When you reach this point with IBS it's actually a cause for celebration, as it means your symptoms have disappeared to the point that you've lost an everpresent motivation for preventing attacks. Out of sight means out of mind sometimes, and this can lead to indulgences that exceed your hard-won confidence.

It's times like these that cheeseburgers and fries have your name written all over them. You think you've been doing so great that surely you don't need to keep slugging down Citrucel every day. You've been so busy lately that even though you enjoy your daily meditation or morning aerobics, you've been missing them because so many other things have you pressed for time. Plus, you feel sure that staying up late to watch that movie tonight won't hurt you. You'll just be a little short on sleep tomorrow but everything will still be okay—after all, you've got your IBS under control.

Then the attack hits you. Once you've recovered you probably follow the same drill I do: kick yourself for being so dumb, for not knowing better, for bringing this misery on yourself. Well, you're allowed a little self-beratement, but it's better to simply give yourself a break. Every single person with IBS has fallen off the wagon, no matter how long they've had the disorder or how successfully they usually manage it. Nobody's perfect, and I'd bet you probably do a terrific job most of the time at giving a one hundred percent effort towards symptom management. Who wouldn't get tired of the constant vigilance this can require? Even ingrained habits that no longer require any real effort to follow can still suffer the occasional lapse.

I've certainly had my struggles in this regard. I've known for more than fifteen years that coffee is a guaranteed trigger for me, and since I don't particularly care for it and never developed the habit of drinking it, I usually avoid it with ease. Then last summer Starbucks came out with frozen raspberry mocha chip Frappucinos, and I found myself unable to resist. My train of thought went something like this: "Surely just a small cup will be okay. I don't think my stomach is *that* empty. Plus I've been doing so well lately. It just looks unbelievably yummy. My friends are all having one. I'm sure I'll be fine…" I drink the whole Frappucino and less than an hour later my thoughts have changed to, "Oh dear God what have I done to myself? Oh no...."

I haven't met anyone else with IBS who doesn't have a similar story to tell. So once again, take comfort in knowing that you're not alone here. Everyone, at some time or another, finds themselves simply unable to resist tempting triggers or failing to do what's necessary to keep stress at bay. This is why it's essential that you have a good support system in place, as these people can help keep you on the straight and narrow when you're inclined to indulge unwisely. They will also be there to give you the care and understanding you need when, despite your best efforts, your IBS flares.

Although the only person who can truly manage your IBS is you, it's crucial to have this support system of friends, family members, and even co-workers. You are having to deal with a serious medical problem on a daily basis through a wide variety of lifestyle modifications, and it is just too tough to do this without the help and understanding of the people closest to you. It's even worse to try and manage an illness like IBS if you're forced to do so in spite of people who deny, minimize, or refuse to accommodate the problem and its restrictions on your life. So if your support system is less than rock-solid, it may be time to take stock of the situation.

How do family members and friends help you cope? Do they help you? If not, why not? What about employers or teachers? Co-workers? Do they really understand what you need from them to be able to manage your symptoms? Do they know and appreciate the IBS dietary requirements? Do they realize the time you require for your stress management program? Are they sympathetic to your needs in general?

If you're not so happy with the answers to those questions, and you don't quite feel that you do have all the support you need, don't hesitate to speak up. Try just sitting down with the people closest to you and discussing the issue. Odds are they truly want to help you and that some of the things you've told them have simply slipped their minds (you might want to refresh their memories with the issues you covered for them back in Week 4).

Try to take into account how difficult it can be for someone who actually has IBS to remember all the factors they need to address in order to control their symptoms—imagine how tricky it is for someone else to have perfect recall on the subject. Even though I've had this disorder since childhood, my friends and family still occasionally offer me foods I cannot eat, because they simply can't remember all the details of my diet. What matters more to me here is the fact that they never fail to ask first whether or not I can eat something, instead of just assuming that I can and having no alternatives available. This is the type of consideration I truly need and appreciate, not necessarily perfect recall on their part of all the dietary guidelines I follow. My husband, on the other hand, knows my diet and other symptom management strategies inside and out right down to the smallest details, and he is a vigilant ally for me in this matter (sometimes even remembering things that slip my mind, like taking my Fibercon tablets before a restaurant meal). I think the difference is simply that he has lived with me and seen me every day, for every single meal, for the past decade. To expect that type of IBS familiarity from my friends and family would be spectacularly unfair.

Your own friends and family probably need some occasional reminders about what IBS is and what you have to do to manage it. Letting them know how genuinely important their support is to you will give them a strong motive to come through for you in the future in every way you need. Reminding them about specific concerns as they arise (could they have baked potato chips instead of fried ones at their picnic? you can't short yourself on sleep so perhaps that early morning appointment could be rescheduled for a later time?) will ensure that your IBS-related needs gradually become ingrained upon them.

If, on the other hand, you must repeatedly deal with someone who simply cannot get it through their head that controlling IBS requires some special considerations, you can either tell them point-blank how much they frustrate you and why, or you can give up and bow out of the relationship altogether. Your course of action will probably depend on your own personality as well as the exact role this person plays in your life (sister versus boss, for instance), but either way the important thing is that you deal with the situation. It is too detrimental to suffer ongoing stress from an uncaring person in your life. You do not need them to maintain control over your IBS (you can do that just fine without them, thank you very much), and there is no point in repeatedly explaining the problem to someone who refuses to listen. Simply cut them out of your life, see them only under circumstances you control, or expect absolutely nothing from them in terms of concern and compassion. If you just assume they'll fail to accommodate your needs they have no power to harm you. Hopefully, your experience with this type of person will be limited—or, better still, non-existent. You're much more likely to find that friends, family members, and co-workers are willing and happy to help you if you simply remind them of your needs as necessary, and express sincere appreciation for their efforts on your behalf.

## IN A SENTENCE:

> *Let the people closest to you know that you appreciate the efforts they make to help you deal with IBS, even when an attack flares due to an indulgence on your part, but don't hesitate to speak up if you're not getting the consideration you need.*

# MONTH **10**

*learning from living*

## task list

1. **CONSIDER HOW MUCH TIME AND ATTENTION (IF ANY) IT'S HEALTHY FOR YOU TO DEVOTE TO IBS OUTSIDE OF YOUR HABITUAL MANAGEMENT STRATEGIES.**

2. **IF YOU'D LIKE TO KEEP CURRENT, CHECK IN WEEKLY WITH INTERNET IBS BOARDS AND HEALTH NEWS SITES.**

3. **CHECK BOOKSTORES AND LIBRARIES FOR NEW IBS LITERATURE.**

# Keep Current with IBS Research— But Only If You Want To

**HOPEFULLY YOU'RE** now well beyond the point of having to think about IBS every day. In fact, once you've got your symptoms under control and have gained the confidence of ongoing good health, it can be counter-productive to spend too much time thinking about the problem. After all, if the impact of IBS on your life is now minimal, so should the time you spend worrying about it. You've surely got better things to concern yourself with.

However, it is always a good idea to keep your eyes and ears open for news about IBS. Since it is considered a lifelong problem, and the underlying dysfunction may unfortunately always be there, you'll probably want to keep yourself well-informed and up-to-date for no other reason than the off chance that a true cure is someday discovered. In fact, because IBS is finally being properly researched, new medications are being developed, and alternative therapies are being tested, there is actually quite a lot of potential for breaking news on the subject. If it has a positive effect on your life to spend a little time dwelling on the subject of IBS, then keep yourself informed of clinical trials, research studies, and general news reports. Make it a habit to look for new books on IBS whenever you're in the library or bookstore, pay attention to information that others in your support group offer, and consider the internet your best tool for keeping current.

You can easily follow the health news headlines through Reuters or AP at many Web sites (including *yahoo, cnn,* and *about*). GI health stories break on a regular basis and you can investigate further into any reports that apply to your situation. Become a member of the International Foundation for Functional Gastrointestinal Disorders (IFFGD), a nonprofit education and research organization whose mission is to inform, assist, and support people affected by functional gastrointestinal disorders. A twenty-five-dollar annual individual membership fee will get you a subscription to *Participate,* their quarterly newsletter. This publication offers the latest research, care, and treatment information for IBS as well as a Reader's Exchange section, which is a regular forum for IFFGD members to share experiences and information. Membership also grants you preferred access to their library of information, and you will be kept up-to-date about IFFGD events, awareness programs, clinical trials, and education programs. Join at *www.iffgd.org.*

Another great option is to check in regularly with the Internet IBS support boards. Try *www.helpforibs.com/messageboards/* (the Bulletin Board section) and *www.ivillage.com* (you have to search a little but it's worth the effort—look under boards, all-health, digestive disorders, IBS). Follow *www.eatingforibs.com* for the latest IBS dietary information and to track IBS publicity efforts.

On the other hand, if you have successfully adjusted your life to control your IBS and are now feeling happy and healthy, and not particularly (or even remotely) interested in continuing to immerse yourself in the subject, then don't. You have truly conquered a health problem when you are able to completely forget about it. If you've reached that point with your IBS it may well have more negative than positive consequences to make the effort of keeping the problem in mind. Personally, I have thought more about IBS these past several years, due to research for books on the topic, than I had in the entire previous decade of living with the disorder. While it was interesting to learn of new discoveries in the field, it was not necessarily to the benefit of my health to be thinking every day about a physical problem that directly affected me—particularly one that carried the baggage of awful past experiences, pain, and suffering. I had long ago found a healthy way to live a happy life through the ingrained habits of controlling my IBS through diet and stress management, and to give the disorder little to no thought beyond that. Becoming immersed in studying the problem gave it pre-eminence in my life once again—not a good thing. So I've decided that from now on regular but cursory glances at IBS news stories are enough to keep me up-to-date without taking more time or thought on the subject than I'm willing to spend. For me, this strikes the right point between being informed and becoming over-involved. Find your own balance in this matter and disregard how others feel on the subject. This is an area where personal preferences are the only ones that matter. Peace of mind is your priority, not whether it takes attention to IBS or the lack thereof to attain it.

## IN A SENTENCE:

> *Keep yourself informed of clinical trials, research studies, and breaking news on IBS, but only if you find this helpful instead of stressful.*

*task list*

1. TAKE A COOKING CLASS WITH AN ETHNIC, VEGETARIAN, OR HEALTH-CONSCIOUS FOCUS.

2. EXPLORE A NEW ETHNIC MARKET (ASIAN, INDIAN, HISPANIC) EACH WEEK.

3. TRY SOME UNUSUAL AND APPEALING INGREDIENTS OR READY-TO-EAT FOODS FROM A HEALTH FOOD STORE.

4. CHECK OUT ETHNIC AND HEALTHY ALTERNATIVE COOKBOOKS FROM THE LIBRARY.

5. PLAN A FULL MEAL FROM A NEW CUISINE AND SHARE THE ADVENTURE WITH FAMILY OR FRIENDS.

# Feeling Adventurous... and Hungry?

**YOU SHOULD** have your diet well under control out of daily habit by now. You're probably familiar with categories of foods to the point of being able to identify fats, soluble fiber, and insoluble fiber in your sleep. Because it can be challenging to learn how to eat safely for IBS, many people gain control of their diet initially by simply limiting the variety of their meals and snacks to a select few tried-and-true favorites. While this is practical and a good way to begin to gain control over food-related attacks, these limitations should not become habitual. In addition to being really dull, any strictly limited diet carries long-term risks in that you need to eat a wide variety of foods in order to obtain essential vitamins and nutrients. In general, the more varied your diet is, the healthier overall you will be. Now that you're an old pro at following the IBS dietary guidelines, it's time to get out of any ruts you feel you're in and explore some delicious new options for cooking and eating safely.

The vast ethnic diversity of markets, cookbooks, and restaurants in America is an absolute godsend for those of us living with IBS who also live to eat (and I am unabashedly first in line here). If you've always wanted to explore a new cuisine, take an off-beat cooking class, or play with the unusual ingredients that entice you at health food stores and ethnic markets, consider IBS a license to experiment.

An easy way to start is to choose an ethnic cuisine (from your favorite restaurant, perhaps?) that you like but wish you were more familiar with—then just roll up your sleeves and prepare to dive in. Find a mouth-watering cookbook or two at the library or bookstore and choose several especially enticing recipes to try first. Take an inventory of your kitchen and note any special cookware required for your new culinary adventure, and make a grocery list of all the ingredients you need. Then head out to a local ethnic market and let the fun begin.

For many ethnic cuisines, it can be handy to have bamboo steamers, a mortar and pestle, rolling pin, hand-hammered wok, a ginger grater, rice steamer, and small ramekins for dipping sauces. You may need special grill pans, bake ware, or prep tools as well. For a splurge, especially if you know you'll be turning to this cuisine often, consider getting ethnic serving bowls, plates, flatware or chopsticks, and so on, to add an extra flourish to your meals. As an aside here, if you've adapted the herbal tea strategies from Month 2, ethnic markets (particularly Asian) offer a treasure trove of special teapots in all sizes, cups, and strainers, in an variety of gorgeous glazes, colors, and patterns. These can add a small touch of luxury to your daily tea habit and turn mere routine into a genuine pleasure.

Once you have all your kitchen tools, head to the food aisles and prepare to stock up—and keep your eye out for special treats to try as well. Give yourself plenty of time to shop so you're able to explore the market in depth. Investigate unusual ingredients that intrigue you, and ask for help if you have questions. I've had great luck getting cooking tips and advice from other customers at ethnic markets—they're often surprised and amused by my questions, but always flattered by the interest in their culture and happy to help. So if something makes you curious, remember that there's bound to be someone in the market who can recommend a use for that herb you're wondering about, or tell you how to best cook the different types of noodles you're eyeing. Feel free to really splurge on these trips, and remember to take your new cookbooks with you to the market. They'll be invaluable when you find an item that looks appealing but wasn't on your shopping list (I guarantee this will happen), as you'll be able to immediately look for a recipe that uses that ingredient. Until you're familiar with your new cuisine you might likely bring home a few things you wind up feeding to the dog, but it's worth taking chances here because you'll also discover fabulous new staples, seasonings, and delicacies. After all, if you don't try something for the first time you'll never know how much you might love it.

Once you're all set with the necessary equipment and ingredients, set aside the blocks of time you need to cook your chosen recipes without being rushed. You're trying something new here, with techniques and foods that may be unfamiliar. Allow yourself the leisure of cooking your meal without racing to finish, so that the experience itself is a fun process of discovery, not a hurried chore. You might even want to devote an entire weekend or a set day of each week to ethnic cooking, so that it becomes an ongoing project and you have the chance to try a wide variety of different recipes. As you take the time to learn and experiment (and eat!) you'll gradually discover exactly which dishes and flavors you prefer, and this will give you a direction to follow as you explore your new cuisine in increasing depth.

On a personal note, IBS is actually a part of what led to my love of ethnic food, and it was also a contributing factor to my interest in cooking in general. Pursuing avenues outside the limited high-fat, meat-and-dairy mainstream American food choices, taking control of what I ate by learning how to prepare it myself, and familiarizing myself with recipes and ingredients, all allowed me to begin the dietary management of my symptoms at a young age. While it's difficult to feel grateful in any way for having IBS, I honestly don't know if I would have explored these subjects to

# Special Treats from Ethnic Markets

**IF YOU** haven't spent much (or any) time in ethnic markets before, you are in for a fun time and some great food. One of my favorite things about all of these markets is the wide variety of unusual, IBS-safe, and delicious ready-to-eat treats they offer. Some are pre-packaged but others are often made fresh each day by the shopkeepers themselves. Here's a list of my favorite ethnic goodies, with a few special ingredients included as well:

## CHINESE AND SOUTHEAST ASIAN

Frozen dim sum dumplings or buns (veggie, seafood, chicken, or bean—just steam them)

Shrimp and veggie uncooked egg rolls (just bake until crispy)

Raised rice cakes (in the bakery section—they're white, soft, spongy, slightly sweet)

Steamed rice and beans in banana leaves (ready to eat)

Banana and rice cakes

Shrimp and scallion noodles (just steam)

Tofu pudding (if you can find it fresh it will come with ginger syrup—heavenly!)

Mango pudding

Snack-pack sizes of soy milk (perfect for lunches and kids)

Fresh fortune cookies

Herbal teas

Dried mango

Flavored soy sauces (stick to Healthy Boy or Lee Kum Kee brands, and try mushroom)

Large grain tapioca pearls (fun for puddings)

Mu-shu pancakes

## JAPANESE

Edamame (fresh whole soybeans, now widely available frozen either in their pods or already shelled—just steam and eat)

Amazake (a naturally sweet, non-fat, non-dairy rice shake—I could live on them!)

Furikake (flavorful sprinkles for rice—often with sesame seeds and sea-weed)

Green teas of every variety

Mochi (rice cakes, fresh or frozen)

Seaweed salads

Soy ice cream

Sushi rolls to-go

Seasoned dried squid (a snack you'll either love or hate)

Packets of instant miso soup (just add boiling water)
Soy-flavored rice crackers (fat-free)

## KOREAN
Kim bap (a Korean, vegetarian sushi rice roll)
Panchan (the "little dishes" of the Korean table, from seasoned vegetables to beans to fish, which make a wonderful meal served with nothing more than lots of steamed rice)
Roasted corn and barley teas (very unique and delicious)
Powdered honey (great for drinks and sprinkling on cereals)

## MIDDLE EASTERN
Fresh pita bread
Lavash (a flat bread)
Fresh hummus
Stuffed grape leaves (make sure there's no meat in them)
Fresh baba ganoush (an eggplant spread)
Fresh tabouli (a couscous salad)
Apricot leather
Pomegranate syrup (great for chicken marinades)
Preserved lemons (delicious to stew with fish, couscous, or vegetable dishes)
Rose preserves (use like jam)
Large grain couscous

## INDIAN
Fresh or frozen naan, paratha, or kulcha breads
Canned ready-to-eat lentil and vegetarian dishes (check for fat content)
Mango nectar
Pappadams (crispy round flatbreads—just broil until they bubble)
Chutneys of every variety
Chai tea
Rose flower water and orange flower water (a very special touch for fruit salads and for baking)
Fresh almonds or pistachios for baking (of much higher quality than in most grocery stores)

## HISPANIC
Horchatas (rice or almond drinks with lime and cinnamon)
Fresh corn tortillas
Fresh tamales (check for no meat or cheese)
Dried fruit leathers (apricot and other flavors)
Passion fruit purée (delicious in drinks)
Mexican cinnamon (add it to safe chocolate dessert recipes or fruit breads)
Epazote (a dried herb to cook with beans to reduce their gassiness)
Pepitas (green pumpkin seeds, delicious when finely ground in seafood sauces)

such a great degree without that additional motivation. For most of my life now much of my free time has revolved around ethnic foods, cookbooks, and restaurants, and this has brought me a great deal of joy, good health, and even a profession in the field. I am thankful for this, even if I would have preferred to have a little less incentive along the way.

As you immerse yourself in ethnic cuisines and broaden your food horizons, consider inviting friends or family over for a casual meal to share your new creations. Do make it clear up front that this is something different and that adventurous tastes are required. You might also note that patience for the cook will be much appreciated, as you may not always get perfect results from your first efforts. You may even want to float the idea with members of your support group of sharing ethnic dishes or dinners, as all of those folks will have the same dietary considerations you do. Hopefully, some will share your culinary interests as well.

If you prefer a little more structure, guidance, or social interaction in your new ethnic explorations, cooking classes may be the perfect option. Check your local community colleges, continuing education classes, and health food stores for interesting upcoming culinary courses. There is likely to be a wide range of ethnic or healthy gourmet options available, and new trends and choices emerge all the time.

If you find a few class descriptions that intrigue you, speak to the instructors before enrolling and ask about the specific foods and cooking methods that will be used. It's a good idea to explain your IBS dietary considerations in a little detail and ask if your needs can be taken into account. If the teachers haven't yet committed to specific recipes, they may well be willing to cook with your dietary requirements in mind. If they already have their classes planned out and can't easily make adjustments, ask them just how adaptable their recipes are—or aren't. Their professional judgment in this matter will be important, but form your own opinions as well, because by this point you are likely to be much more knowledgeable about and experienced in making the types of dietary substitutions required for IBS than a Michelin-starred chef. Some things to consider along these lines: if something is supposed to be deep fried, can you skillet-fry it in a nonstick pan with cooking oil instead? if dairy is called for, can you substitute soy or rice equivalents? what if you used two egg whites to replace each whole egg? how much oil can just be eliminated from the recipes altogether?

If you don't find satisfactory answers to these questions, or if you discover that most of the class recipes will be near-impossible to safely modify (pork chimichangas or tempura, say), accept that this particular course isn't going to fit the IBS bill. Don't give up, just keep looking. There isn't a country in the world with no culinary specialties you can eat, so don't even feel that you have to abandon your ethnic first choice. Try looking specifically for low-fat emphasis classes (this is crucial for Mediterranean and classical French food), or ones that lean toward seafood and vegan dishes. You may even find an instructor willing to tailor an upcoming class to some of the IBS requirements so that you can participate. At the very least, it won't hurt to ask.

Another option for exploring new and unusual culinary choices is your local health food market. There are many great national chains now that are just as huge, and offer as wide a variety of foods, as standard grocery stores. In addition, these markets also have a tremendous range of bulk foods, organic products, soy foods, fresh baked breads, and a staggering variety of vegetarian convenience choices.

A great place to start is the freezer section, where you'll find so many low-fat vegan versions of standard American junk food products your heart will sing. You can stock up on everything from hotdogs to chicken wings, cheddar cheese slices to pizza pockets, and they will all be low-fat, meat-, dairy-, and preservative-free. They're quite likely to be delicious too, though you'll find the occasional item that just doesn't make the cut. A fun splurge is tofu or rice ice cream and fudgesicles (check the fat content).

For something new and interesting, head to the bulk food aisles and check out the huge variety of grains, flours, soy substitutes, pastas, and more. (Don't forget a detour down the herb counter to stock up— inexpensively—on your favorite teas, such as peppermint, anise, or chamomile.) Most health food markets have free pamphlets in their bulk sections that give information about all the items, cooking instructions, serving suggestions, and nutritional analyses. You can try everything from blue cornmeal pancake mix (make with soy milk and egg whites) to instant vegan chili, to hummus mix (just add water) in the bulk section, and I have yet to try a single product like this that wasn't just delicious. There are also many unusual grains (try quinoa and the native rices), whole barley (much more flavorful than pearl), oat groats, couscous (cooks in just minutes), soba noodles (made from buckwheat flour), and dozens of other choices.

Get a small trial bag of everything that appeals to you, and come back another day to stock up on your new favorites.

Bulk aisles also offer a wide range of specialty dried fruits great for baking, vegetable broth for soup-making, soy protein products such as TVP (the perfect ground meat substitute), unrefined sugars, and other invaluable ingredients for expanding your healthy gourmet cooking options.

Next, take a quick trip down the sauce aisle, and look for flavorful shortcuts to let you season standard fare (rice stir fries, baked chicken breasts, grilled fish) quickly and deliciously. As long as your choices are low-fat, you can go to town here and find Thai, Mexican, Indian, Ethiopian, Greek, and a dozen other choices in dips, salsas, chutneys, marinades, and more. Health food stores offer a wealth of high-flavor, low-fat (and preservative/artificial ingredient-free) sauces, which will let you expand your culinary creativity without much time and effort at all in the kitchen. These ready-made items provide a great way to try some of the flavors of ethnic fare without going to all the effort and expense of finding and buying the unfamiliar ingredients and specialty kitchen equipment needed to cook an authentic dish from scratch. Once you find a new taste you like, you can take the additional steps needed to making home-cooked meals from that cuisine with confidence.

The only precautions you need to take in any of your ethnic explorations are to follow the IBS dietary guidelines you learned way back in your first few days and weeks, and which you surely know by heart by now. Keep those in mind, and you can eat safely and deliciously from all around the world—right in your own kitchen. Bon appetit!

**IN A SENTENCE:**

> *Consider IBS an invitation to try delicious new choices for cooking and eating safely by exploring ethnic markets, cookbooks, classes, and health food markets.*

*task list*

1. TAKE PEN TO PAPER AND LIST THE MOST SUCCESSFUL STRATEGIES YOU'VE FOUND FOR CONTROLLING YOUR IBS.

2. NOTE ANY ONGOING PROBLEMS IN YOUR ROUTINE, TIMES WHEN SYMPTOMS TEND TO FLARE, AND ALL AREAS WHERE YOU KNOW YOU STILL NEED IMPROVEMENTS.

3. LOOK TO THE FUTURE AND ANTICIPATE ANY PROBLEMATIC EVENTS, LIFESTYLE CHANGES, OR DISRUPTIONS IN YOUR LIFE, AND MAKE PLANS NOW TO DEAL WITH THEM.

4. DETERMINE THE BEST WAYS TO MAINTAIN YOUR SUCCESSFUL STRATEGIES, SHORE UP ANY WEAKNESSES, AND BEGIN NEW PRACTICES THAT ARE LIKELY TO HELP YOU.

# Review and Reflect

CONGRATULATIONS! YOU'VE just survived your first year with an officially diagnosed case of Irritable Bowel Syndrome. Of course, the odds are you've actually been suffering from the problem for quite a bit longer, but this just makes a warm pat on the back even more well-deserved. So go ahead, it's time for a little self-congratulatory indulgence. You've accomplished a heck of a lot in just a year, from major dietary changes to stress management practices. Hopefully you've also tried some alternative therapies along the way, found a sympathetic support group, joined the campaign for media attention to IBS, and learned to cook some new ethnic recipes.

How do you feel about what you've accomplished? Are you where you hoped you'd be at the end of this year? Did you exceed your expectations or are you disappointed with your progress? How much greater is your control over IBS now than when you were first diagnosed?

Take a fair assessment of what strategies have worked the best for you. Are there any options you still haven't tried? Now is the time to give them a shot, whatever they may be. Decide which approaches delivered the best results for you—diet? medication? yoga? hypnotherapy?—and what you can do to maintain your improvements. Take a long look at strategies you've so far shied away from and ask yourself if you should give them a decent try.

As you evaluate your first year of living with IBS, try to spot the weaknesses in your lifestyle management plan. When do attacks flare despite your best efforts? Is there an identifiable pattern to this problem that will help you solve it? Are there any approaches that do work for you but that you have trouble maintaining consistently? Now is the time to take the success you've reached so far to a higher level, and figure out a way to make things even better for you. Allocate the time, effort, money, or other resources necessary to gain further improvements, and make a commitment to taking the steps needed to achieve your goals. As always, your health should be a priority. You are worth it.

Look ahead as well as behind, and consider what's on the horizon for the upcoming year. Put a plan into effect to maintain the various lifestyle modifications that have given you the best results. Reinforce these most successful habits to ensure they become a permanent part of your life. Take it for granted that challenges to your diet and stress management will surely arise—that's life—but be reassured that dealing with them will be easier now that you've gained confidence borne of experience and success. Scrutinize your future and see if you spot any potential problems arising with your IBS. If you do, start now to do whatever it takes to stay in charge of your health, your life, and your happiness.

To gain a little perspective, review this book from the introductory chapters on. Realize how far you've come and how much you've learned. If you can take a real step back from your situation and objectively consider the entire past year, I hope you'll see a silver lining to the IBS cloud. In truth, following the dietary strategy, stress management routines, and alternative therapies that allow you to minimize the impact of your IBS should also have a significant positive influence on your life as a whole. Each of these practices will give you better physical, mental, and emotional health overall, with long-term benefits far beyond the realm of your GI tract. Gaining control of IBS through lifestyle modifications carries the welcome side effects of lowering your risk for many chronic and fatal illnesses, helps to slow the aging process, and will force you to find a healthy balance in your life. You'll have developed the habit of paying close attention to your body along the way, and you probably will forever after, which will keep you informed and aware of your health and what you need to take care of it.

You'll know your IBS is totally under control when you can genuinely view the disorder as, while not exactly a blessing in disguise (that would be pushing it), but a part of your life that, in the end, resulted in better health and happiness for you overall. Now, put this book down, and go take a well-deserved break. Because the one thing above all else I hope you've realized this past year is that while IBS may be a part of your life, it doesn't have to run it.

**IN A SENTENCE:**

> *Assess what strategies have been most successful for controlling your IBS, try to find the areas where you could further reduce your triggers, and congratulate yourself on all you have learned and accomplished this past year.*

# Glossary

**ALLODYNIA:** Pain perceived in non-sensory pathways. Allodynia is involved in the development of **visceral** hypersensitivity that characterizes IBS.

**ANAL VERGE:** The internal part of the **anus** is called the anal canal. It's a cylinder of tissue about two to three centimeters (one inch) long, and the patch of external skin immediately around the opening of the anus is known as the anal margin. The point where the anal canal and anal margin meet one another is called the anal verge.

**ANUS:** The last part of the gastrointestinal tract, the anus is at the extreme end of the rectum. It's composed of a sphincter muscle which relaxes to allow the passage of fecal material.

**COLON:** The colon (large intestine) has six major parts: cecum, ascending colon, transverse colon, descending colon, sigmoid colon, and rectum. The total length is approximately five feet in an adult. The colon is responsible for forming, storing, and expelling waste matter.

The **cecum** is the pouch-like beginning of the colon in the right lower quadrant of the abdomen (the appendix extends off the cecum).

The **ascending colon** is the next part of the organ, which starts in the right lower quadrant of the abdomen and ends at the transverse colon in the right upper quadrant of the abdomen.

The **transverse colon** is the third division of the large intestine. It communicates with the ascending colon and the descending colon.

The **descending colon** is the fourth portion of the large intestine. It communicates with the transverse colon above and the rectum below.

The **sigmoid colon** is an extension of mobile descending colon, and it connects to the descending colon above and the rectum below.

The **rectum** is the last portion of the large intestine. It communicates with the sigmoid colon above and the anus below.

**GASTROCOLIC REFLEX:** A partly **neurogenic** process in which there is an increase in colonic motility, triggered by the stomach upon eating. After-meal deviations from the normal gastrocolic reflex muscle contraction patterns lead to the altered bowel habits of IBS.

**GERD:** Gastroesophageal Reflux Disease. GERD is a digestive disorder that affects the lower esophageal sphincter (the muscle connecting the esophagus with the stomach). Gastroesophageal refers to the stomach and esophagus. Reflux means to flow back or return. Therefore, GERD is the return of the stomach's contents back up into the esophagus. GERD frequently causes heartburn or acid indigestion.

**HYPERALGESIA:** A lower pain threshold. Hyperalgesia is involved in the development of **visceral** hypersensitivity that characterizes IBS.

**INSOLUBLE FIBER:** Insoluble fiber is a subclass of dietary fiber. Insoluble fiber is considered a "noncarbohydrate carbohydrate" since the components that make up insoluble fiber are lignins, cellulose, and hemicelluloses. All of these compounds form the structural parts of plants and do not readily dissolve in water and are not metabolized by intestinal bacteria.

**NEUROGENIC:** Originating in the nervous system.

**NEUROLOGICAL:** Having to do with the nerves or the nervous system.

**NEUROLOGIC INNERVATION:** Stimulation of the nerves or nervous system.

**NEUROTRANSMITTER:** A chemical which conveys or inhibits nerve impulses.

**PATHOPHYSIOLOGY:** Functional changes associated with or resulting from disease or injury.

**PERISTALSIS:** The wavelike muscular contractions of the digestive tract by which its contents are forced onward.

**SEROTONIN:** A biochemical messenger and regulator, found primarily in the central nervous system, gastrointestinal tract, and blood platelets. Serotonin mediates several important physiological functions including gastrointestinal motility. Multiple receptor families explain the broad physiological actions and distribution of serotonin.

**SOLUBLE FIBER:** Soluble fiber is a subclass of dietary fiber. Food compounds that dissolve or swell when put into water are called soluble fibers. These compounds include pectins, gums, mucilages, and some hemicelluloses. They're found inside and around plant cells.

**SOMATIC:** Of, relating to, or affecting the body, especially as distinguished from the mind or the environment.

**VISCERAL:** Relating to the soft internal abdominal organs, particularly the intestines. Colloquially, "guts."

# Acknowledgments

**MY THANKS** to my editor, Matthew Lore, for cajoling out of me a book I really didn't think I could write, but am very glad I did. Thank you to Ling Lucas and Janis Donnaud, my stellar agents. Thanks to Sue McCloskey, Ghadah Alrawi, Pauline Neuwirth, Howard Grossman, and everyone else who contributed to the production and design of the book. My eternal gratitude to all those who shared their personal stories for this book, including Ann G., Diane Feierabend, Shawn Eric Case, Analy Alfonso, Kit Gorrell, Monique Spencer, Melissa D. Godwin, Jeffrey Roberts, and Mindy Helm. A special thanks to Michael Mahoney, for his time, generosity, and devotion to the IBS cause. Thank you as well to my wonderful family and friends for their endless patience, support, good humor, love, and understanding.

# Index